Ultrasound and Fetal Growth

PROGRESS IN OBSTETRIC
AND GYNECOLOGICAL
SONOGRAPHY SERIES

SERIES EDITOR: ASIM KURJAK

Ultrasound and
Fetal Growth

Edited by

J. M. CARRERA, G. P. MANDRUZZATO
and K. MAEDA

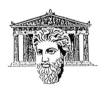

The Parthenon Publishing Group
International Publishers in Medicine, Science & Technology

NEW YORK   LONDON

Library of Congress
Cataloging-in-Publication Data
Ultrasound and fetal growth / edited by J. M.
Carrera . . . [et al.].
     p. cm. — (Progress in obstetric and
gynecological sonography series)
  Includes bibliographical references and
index.
   ISBN 1-85070-618-2
   1. Fetus—Growth. 2. Ultrasonics in obstetrics.
I. Carrera, José María, 1937–   .
II. Series.
   [DNLM: 1. Fetal Growth Retardation—
ultrasonography.
2. Ultrasonography, Prenatal.   WQ 210.5 U47
1999]
RG613.U45   1999
618.3'207543—dc21
DNLM/DLC
for Library of Congress   99-16520
                         C IP

British Library Cataloguing in Publication Data
Ultrasound and fetal growth. – (Progress in
obstetric and gynecological sonography series)
  1. Fetus – Growth 2. Fetus – Ultrasonic imaging
I. Perez Carrera, Jose Manuel
II. Mandruzzato, G. P.
III. Maeda, Kei-ichiro
612.6'47

ISBN 1-85070-618-2

Published in the USA by
The Parthenon Publishing Group Inc.
One Blue Hill Plaza
PO Box 1564, Pearl River
New York 10965, USA

Published in the UK and Europe by
The Parthenon Publishing Group Limited
Casterton Hall, Carnforth
Lancs. LA6 2LA, UK

Copyright © 2001
The Parthenon Publishing Group

Typeset by H&H Graphics, Blackburn, UK
Printed by Bookcraft (Bath) Ltd.,
Midsomer Norton, UK

Contents

List of contributors

J. M. Carrera
Institut Universitari Dexeus
Passeig Bonanova 67
08017 Barcelona
Spain

C. Comas
Institut Universitari Dexeus
Passeig Bonanova 67
08017 Barcelona
Spain

R. Devesa
Institut Universitari Dexeus
Passeig Bonanova 67
08017 Barcelona
Spain

G. D'Ottavio
Istituto per l'Infanza
Via dell'Istria 65/1
Trieste
Italy

R. B. Elejalde
Medical Genetics Institute
4555 West Schroeder Drive, Suite 180
Brown Deer
Wisconsin 53223
USA

K. Maeda
Seirei Hamamatsu General Hospital
Sumiyoshi 2-12-2
Hamamatsu 430
Japan

G. P. Mandruzzato
Istituto per l'Infanza
Via dell'Istria 65/1
Trieste
Italy

C. Mortera
Institut Universitari Dexeus
Passeig Bonanova 67
08017 Barcelona
Spain

A. Muñoz
Institut Universitari Dexeus
Passeig Bonanova 67
08017 Barcelona
Spain

M. Torrents
Institut Universitari Dexeus
Passeig Bonanova 67
08017 Barcelona
Spain

Color plates

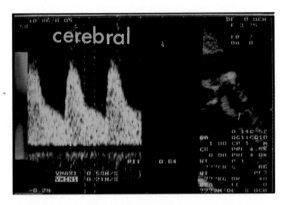

Color plate A   Middle cerebral artery waveform. Low pulsatility index. Vasodilatation of cerebral blood vessels

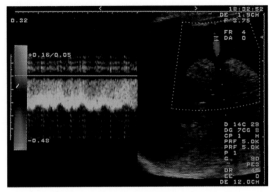

Color plate B   Venous pulsation in umbilical vein

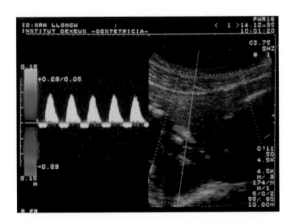

Color plate C   Reverse diastolic flow in umbilical artery

Preface

Alterations of fetal growth, widely explained in this book, still constitute a challenge for the diagnostic capacity and clinical sense of obstetricians. Only a multidisciplinary approach to the problem will permit understanding of the causes and pathogenic mechanisms that are involved and, at the same time, achieve a decrease in perinatal morbidity and mortality.

From a diagnostic point of view, the use of ultrasonography in obstetrics has demonstrated its efficacy in measuring fetal structures and therefore in detecting anomalies of intrauterine growth prenatally. This diagnostic capacity has been extended as new techniques, particularly Doppler and all its variants, have also permitted, with notable success, the study of fetal and placental hemodynamics. The result is that we are in the position not only of determining growth patterns of the fetus but also of checking objective parameters of its health and following up possible hemodynamic deterioration.

This book, with all its limitations, conveys the current state of the art in this field, expressing current attitudes and emphasizing a practical orientation.

The Editors of the book wish to thank Professor Asim Kurjak for his friendship and trust in asking them to compile the book. They also express their gratitude to the contributors and collaborators of the three Obstetrics and Gynecological Departments (Institut Universitari Dexeus of Barcelona, Istituto per l'Infanza of Trieste and Seirei Hamamatsu General Hospital) who have made it possible.

J. M. Carrera
G. P. Mandruzzato
K. Maeda

Fetal growth characteristics

1

J. M. Carrera, R. B. Elejalde and R. Devesa

INTRODUCTION

'Growth' is usually defined as the process whereby the body mass of a living being increases in size as a result of the increase in number (hyperplasia) and size (hypertrophy) of its cells and intracellular matrix. 'Development', on the other hand, should be understood as the process by which organs and their regulatory mechanisms gradually assume their functions in living beings. Broadly speaking, the term 'growth' is preferred when referring to measurable anatomical changes; 'development' is used to refer to the gradual acquisition of certain specific physiological functions.

The fetal growth rate is mainly determined by the intrinsic potential of fetal growth, which is primarily genetically controlled ('genetic factor'). However, the influence of this genetic factor is considerably modified by two other intrauterine regulating factors of fetal growth, the 'hormone factor', fetal and growth promotoring, and the 'environmental factor', maternal and usually growth restraining.

The fetal growth curve during gestation and ultimately the weight at birth are, therefore, the result of the interaction between growth restraining and promoting factors. The human fetus may be considered to be the result of the interaction of its genetic potential, its possibility of 'being', and the circumstances surrounding its attempt to 'be' – the environment, which limits or favors it.

The genetic factor, which imposes fairly narrow limits of variability, dominates during the first half of pregnancy, whereas hormone and environmental factors exert their greatest influence during the second half of pregnancy, resulting in a widening of the limits of variability in fetal growth and development. For this reason the fetal growth rate is not constant during pregnancy but rather shows a progressive, sustained transition from the exponential rate (in the first weeks of pregnancy) to the linear rate (in late pregnancy)[1].

ANTHROPOMETRIC STUDIES

Intrauterine growth characteristics can be studied by means of: first, neonatal anthropometry, which is a simple and reliable method that allows the construction of weight–gestational-age curves of normality and discrimination of neonates undergoing pathological variations; and second, fetal anthropometry, which has been developed according to the possibility of assessing the size and growth of different fetal parameters using radiological or ultrasonographic techniques.

Theoretically, anthropometric studies can be carried out following four study designs:

(1) Cross-sectional studies;

(2) Longitudinal studies;

(3) Longitudinal studies with data interpolation;

(4) Multilevel models.

Cross-sectional studies

In this type of study, each individual is considered on a single occasion. It has the advantage that growth curves for a given population can be constructed in a short period of time, allowing precise focusing on selected variables[2]. Obviously, cross-sections do not permit the same individual or the same group to be followed over time. Despite these limitations, these are the only types of study that can be carried out in the field of neonatal anthropometry since neonates can be weighed or measured only once.

Longitudinal studies

In this case, an individual or a group of individuals undergo a series of measurements at established intervals. Therefore, the time-course of the same population is assessed, whereas different populations are included in cross-sectional studies. This method can be used both in intrauterine and in postnatal anthropometry, in which case measurements are taken through ultrasound or a radiological view of the fetus (fetal biometry). Longitudinal studies are always more difficult to perform than cross-sectional studies (because of problems in attaining similar initial and final sample sizes) and take longer.

Longitudinal studies with data interpolation

Because of the difficulties in obtaining serial follow-up data of a given population without drop-outs or a marked reduction in the number of participants, on many occasions interpolations have to be relied on, in order to fill blank spaces in graphs by mathematical or graphic methods[2].

Multilevel models

Most growth curves available in the literature based on either cross-sectional or longitudinal studies are currently open to criticism. Inadequacies of study design, including inappropriate selection of cases, unclear inclusion and exclusion criteria, small sample size, unreliable gestational ages and, particularly, inefficiency of the individual method applied to construct the regression lines[3,4], are the main reasons argued.

Several authors insist on the usefulness of computer-generated multilevel models in the study of fetal growth[5] based on the current development of computer technology[6,7]. Data of the longitudinal study are stratified into a hierarchy in the structure of the computer design. Two levels, for instance, would be the simplest method: variations among gestational ages of the same fetus (level 1) and variations among fetuses of the same gestational age (level 2), although countless levels might be established by the introduction of other variables.

NEONATAL ANTHROPOMETRY

Although obtaining different neonatal body measurements is feasible, most authors have limited the assessment of intrauterine growth to the following neonatal parameters: weight, height, head circumference and chest circumference.

Weight

All authors agree that fetal weight is the most sensitive indicator of fetal growth and nutrition, since fetal weight is the earliest parameter to be affected by an adverse intrauterine environment. However, for this reason and because of the high variability in birth weight among different human populations[8], it is difficult to obtain a pattern of fetal growth based only on the weight of the fetus, especially since there is a linear relationship between weight at birth and duration of gestation. On the other hand, the construction of tables or curves of normal fetal weight at different weeks of gestation faces several difficulties, the first of which is the fact that data derived from longitudinal studies are unreliable (a fetus or a neonate can be weighed only once, and previous weight variations are unknown). Another important difficulty is related to the fact that weights of fetuses born prematurely cannot be included in the range of normality. Last, comparison of different tables and curves is further complicated by the lack of uniformity in the entry of data.

The first extended curve of fetal growth based on birth weight data was published by Lubchenko and colleagues from Denver (USA)[1] in the form of centiles relating weight and gestational age from 24 to 42 weeks of gestation (Figure 1). Almost simultaneously,

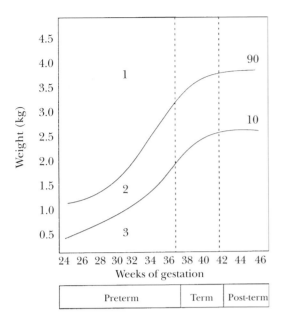

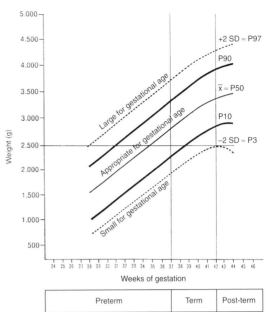

Figure 1 Statistical definitions of weight centiles for gestational age. 1, large for gestational age; 2, appropriate for gestational age; 3, small for gestational age

Figure 2 Relationship between the centile curves of Lubchenko[1] and the curves of Gruenwald[9,10] expressing standard deviations

Gruenwald[9,10] estimated intrauterine growth in the form of standard deviations (Figure 2). Thereafter, other curves constructed according to these two criteria were reported by many authors from different parts of the world. These curves, however, cannot be superimposed, owing to differences in socioeconomic conditions, altitude, racial features, etc. Curves constructed in Spain, France, Italy and Czechoslovakia show fetal weights higher than those of Lubchenko and colleagues[1] (Denver, Colorado, is 1584 m above sea level) which, in turn, are lower than those reported by Swedish authors[11,12].

Most fetal growth curves can be divided into four areas of different fetal growth rates (Figure 3): low rate (up to 16 weeks' gestation with a mean weight gain of ≤ 10 g/week); accelerated rate (between 16 and 26–27 weeks' gestation with a mean weight gain up to 85 g/week); maximal rate (between 28 and 38 weeks' gestation with a mean weight gain of 200 g/week); and decelerated rate (around 37–38 weeks' gestation with a mean weight

gain of 70 g/week). Beyond 42 weeks' gestation, fetal weight shows no variation or negligible increases.

It should be noted that 10% of the weight at term is exclusively reached during the first half of pregnancy, and it is only after the first two trimesters of pregnancy that the fetus acquires one-third of its weight at birth. However, it should be remembered that, during the first half of pregnancy, organogenesis and progressive development and refinement of fetal structures take place.

The most crucial period of fetal life starts about 28 weeks of gestation, coinciding with the maximal slope of fetal weight gain (200 g/week). This means, for example, that in case of premature delivery threat, fetal prognosis largely improves when it is possible to gain time with appropriate therapy.

As noted by Gruenwald[13], all fetal weight curves with the exception of those corresponding to stillborn infants coincide at 38 weeks' gestation, probably because the possibility of error in the gestational age at

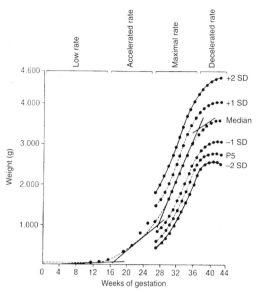

Figure 3 Division of fetal growth curves in four areas: low rate, accelerated rate, maximal rate, decelerated rate

this time is remote. However, differences before this period, which in some cases may be considerable, can be attributed to deficiencies in information or inadequacies of correction.

Height

The first fetal height curves throughout the gestational period were also constructed by Lubchenko and colleagues[1]. As in the case of fetal weight, the fetal height curve shows a moderate sigmoid shape with an ascending trend as gestational age increases.

Head circumference

Head circumference has considerable importance, since it is well known that fetal brain weight is the parameter least affected by intrauterine malnutrition. For this reason, although fetal head circumference is not a reliable index of fetal growth and nutrition, it is a sensitive indicator of gestational age; in some cases, the comparison of this parameter with the remaining indicators of fetal growth

provides useful information. In general, head circumference curves undergo few fluctuations and inflections.

Thoracic diameter

As compared with the literature regarding other fetal growth parameters, references to thoracic diameter are limited. In Spain, this subject has been studied by Alonso and Arizcun[14], who suggested that the lack of references might be related to the greater difficulty in the measurement of this parameter. The so-called mean thoracic diameter, between inspiration and expiration, should be recorded.

FETAL GROWTH PATTERNS

Normal growth patterns

The growth of a fetus with normal genetic and environmental growth factors has the following characteristics[15]:

(1) Both weight and height increases show a linear, constant and dependent pattern.

(2) Each organ and tissue has a different growth rate but the proportion between organs and tissues remains constant.

(3) The measurement of a given organ or tissue allows prediction with acceptable accuracy of the size of other organs or tissues.

(4) Since tables and equations of normality data have been based on data from a sufficiently large population, incorporating variations of the normal population, measurements of all normal individuals will fit within the normal range.

(5) There is a large variation of human fetal growth and dimensions at different gestational ages. This characteristic should be taken into consideration when deciding on the normality or abnormality of a given individual.

Abnormal growth patterns

(1) Weight and height increases are not linear functions and express independent actions. The specific pattern of the abnormality relates in part to the etiology of the pathological process.

(2) As a result of the abnormal growth, the correct proportion of tissues is lost (e.g. normal head accompanied by abnormally short limbs).

(3) The size of an organ cannot be used for predicting dimensions of another organ or tissue, because growth rate becomes independent as a result of the pathogenetic process and the protective mechanisms involved.

(4) If tables or equations of normality data have been obtained from a sufficiently large population to incorporate variations of the normal population, measurements of all abnormal individuals will fit outside the normal range. The distribution of measurements of normal and abnormal fetuses will be markedly different, with a transitional zone in which there is an overlapping of normally small and abnormally small individuals, and of normally large and abnormally large individuals. These transitional zones are very useful in clinical practice since they allow early signs of abnormal growth to be identified.

(5) There is great variation in growth rates and dimensions of abnormal human fetuses at different gestational ages. This feature should be taken into consideration when deciding on the normality or abnormality of a given individual.

(6) Abnormal fetal growth patterns vary widely in relation to etiology.

References

1. Lubchenko LO, Hansman C, Dressler M, Boyd E. Intrauterine growth as estimated from liveborn birth-weight data at 24 to 42 weeks of gestation. *Pediatrics* 1963;32:793–800
2. Carrera JM, Devesa R, Carrera M. Dinámics del crecimiento fetal. In Carrera JM, ed. *Crecimiento Fetal*. Barcelona: Masson, 1997:3–29
3. Royston P, Altman DG. Design and analysis of longitudinal studies of fetal size. *Ultrasound Obstet Gynecol* 1995;6:307–12
4. Royston P. Calculation of unconditional and conditional reference intervals for fetal size and growth from longitudinal measurements. *Stat Med* 1995;14:1417–36
5. Goldstein H. Efficient statistical modelling of longitudinal data. *Ann Hum Biol* 1986;13:129–41
6. Prosser R, Rasbash J, Goldstein H. *ML3 Software for Three-level Analysis. User's Guide for Version 2.* London: Institute of Education, 1991
7. Rasbash J, Woodhouse G. *MLn Command Reference. Version 1.0.* London: Institute of Education, 1995
8. Meredith HC. Body weight at birth of viable human infants: a worldwide comparative treatise. *Hum Biol* 1970;42:217–64
9. Gruenwald P. The fetus in prolonged pregnancy. *Am J Obstet Gynecol* 1964;89:503–9
10. Gruenwald P. Infants of low birth weight among 5000 deliveries. *Pediatrics* 1964;34:157–62
11. Sterky G. Swedish standard curves for intrauterine growth. *Pediatrics* 1970;46:7–8
12. Lindell A. Prolonged pregnancy. *Acta Obstet Gynecol Scand* 1956;35:136–63
13. Gruenwald P. Growth of the human fetus. 1. Normal growth and its variation. *Am J Obstet Gynecol* 1966;94:1112–19
14. Alonso T, Arizcun J. Antropometría perinatal. *Acta Ginecol* 1975;27:449–66
15. Elejalde RB, Elejalde MM. Análisis antropométrico del feto humano in utero. In Carrera JM, ed. *Crecimiento Fetal*. Barcelona: Masson, 1997:189–215

Principles and techniques of fetal ultrasound biometry

2

G. P. Mandruzzato, G. D'Ottavio and J. M. Carrera

BASIC PRINCIPLES

Fetal anthropometry is based on the biometric assessment of different fetal parameters according to which the clinical course of fetal growth can be studied. At present, ultrasonography is the only suitable technique for *in utero* evaluation of fetal anthropometry. Ultrasound scanning permits an accurate estimation to be made of dimensions of different body segments, long bones and particular organs. The availability of normal growth curves and tables for all these structures facilitates, for a properly trained echographer, the follow-up of fetal growth throughout the gestational period as well as the diagnosis of either excessive or defective pathological changes in fetal growth.

However, for fetal ultrasound biometry to be reliable and useful in obstetric practice, the following principles should be taken into account:

(1) 'Size' is a physical dimension that can be measured at a given time. It forms part of the fetal structural ultrasound study. By contrast, 'growth' is a dynamic process that involves size changes over time, so that serial observations are required for its assessment. It forms part of the fetal functional ultrasound study[1].

(2) Fetal echo-biometry requires sufficient ultrasonographic experience and a methodology of meticulous measurement. Errors in the estimation of biometric parameters may lead to completely false conclusions regarding fetal growth.

(3) A reliable knowledge of the gestational age is essential for indicating the usefulness of an ultrasound assessment of fetal growth. In this sense, it is necessary to know which biometric parameters, independent of growth abnormalities, are consistently related to gestational age.

(4) Curves or tables used should be appropriate for the studied population and as far as possible derived from a longitudinal rather than from a cross-sectional study.

(5) For a correct interpretation of curves or tables that correlate gestational age with selected biometric values, it is necessary to know the independent parameter according to which the dependent variable has been studied. The dependent parameter can be estimated or deduced from the former, but not vice versa. In practice, independent variables are placed on the abscissa and dependent variables on the ordinate. Accordingly, different curves should be used for ultrasound assessment of gestational age and fetal growth (Figure 1).

(6) An adequate knowledge of fetal pathophysiology and of predictable growth patterns in different pathological conditions is required for interpretation of biometric data. The correct inter-relationship of the data obtained would be possible only if the echographer were able to elaborate a spatial mental image.

This chapter includes a review of fetal biometry during the first trimester of pregnancy (which would usually allow a

7

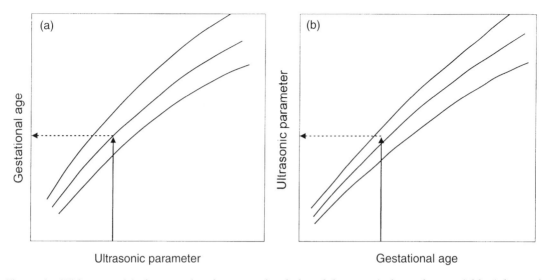

Figure 1 With curve (a) the gestational age can be deduced from an independent variable (ultrasonic parameter), but if the aim is to study fetal growth, the appropriate curve is (b), where the independent variable is gestational age

precise gestational age to be established), followed by a study of segmental fetal biometry, skeletal biometry, biometry of fetal organs, the biometric indices and ultrasonographic calculation of fetal weight.

ULTRASOUND FOR ASSESSMENT OF GESTATIONAL AGE

In order to perform a correct fetal ultrasound biometric study, a fundamental aspect is to know the gestational age as exactly as possible. Early ultrasound examination carried out during the first trimester of pregnancy permits determination of gestational age with remarkable precision on the basis of gestational sac and yolk sac biometry, but especially by assessing the crown–rump length (CRL).

The CRL is a particularly sensitive biometric parameter that can be measured in the early stages of gestation[2]. The only technical limitation is the progressive bending of the embryo, which makes measurements less reliable after weeks 10–12 of gestation. Between weeks 6 and 12 of gestation, there is an exponential increase in CRL, although this increase later appears to be linear (Figure 2). A rough error at early stages consists of adding

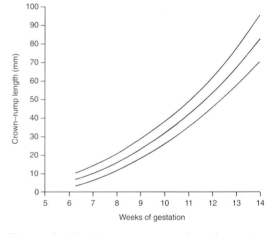

Figure 2 Fetal crown–rump length against gestational age

yolk sac diameter to CRL. The maxium error obtained when calculating this parameter with respect to gestational age is ± 5 days in 95% of cases, because between weeks 6 and 14 fetal growth is rapid and the limits of confidence are very narrow. According to this parameter it would be possible to establish an early assessment of abnormal embryonic growth. CRL can be measured from week 6 of

Table 1 Assessment of gestational age from crown–rump length (CRL). There were no significant differences when results obtained by different authors using either transabdominal or transvaginal transducers were compared

CRL (mm)	Gestational age (weeks)			
	Robinson[2] (transabdominal)	Nelson[3] (transabdominal)	Drumm et al.[4] (transabdominal)	Hadlock et al.[5] (transvaginal)
10	7.0	8.1	6.9	7.1
12	7.4	8.3	7.3	7.4
14	7.7	8.5	7.6	7.7
16	8.0	8.6	7.9	8.0
18	8.3	8.8	8.2	8.3
20	8.5	9.0	8.5	8.6
22	8.8	9.2	8.7	8.9
24	9.0	9.3	9.0	9.1
26	9.3	9.5	9.2	9.4
28	9.5	9.7	9.5	9.6
30	9.7	9.9	9.7	9.9
32	9.9	10.0	9.9	10.1
34	10.0	10.2	10.1	10.3
36	10.3	10.4	10.4	10.5
38	10.5	10.5	10.6	10.7
40	10.7	10.7	10.8	10.9
42	10.8	10.9	11.0	11.1
44	11.0	11.1	11.2	11.2
46	11.2	11.2	11.3	11.4
48	11.4	11.4	11.5	11.6
50	11.5	11.6	11.7	11.7
52	11.7	11.7	11.9	11.9
54	11.8	11.9	12.1	12.0
56	12.0	12.1	12.2	12.2
58	12.1	12.3	12.4	12.3
60	12.3	12.4	12.6	12.5
62	12.4	12.6	12.7	12.6
64	12.6	12.8	12.9	12.8
66	12.7	12.9	13.0	12.9
68	12.9	13.1	13.2	13.1
70	13.0	13.3	13.4	13.2
72	13.1	13.5	13.5	13.4
74	13.3	13.6	13.7	13.5
76	13.4	13.8	13.8	13.7
78	13.5	14.0	14.0	13.8
80	13.7	14.1	14.1	14.0

gestation with the use of transvaginal transducers and from week 7 of gestation using transabdominal transducers.

As shown in Table 1, there are no significant differences when results obtained by different authors using either transabdominal or transvaginal transducers are compared[2–5]. Most authors have not found statistically significant differences according to race or gender[6,7] except for the series of Pedersen[8], who reported a significantly larger CRL in male fetuses than in females (mean value of gender difference: 2 mm).

FETAL ULTRASOUND BIOMETRY FOR EVALUATING FETAL GROWTH

The assessment of fetal growth is an integral part of obstetric management, because fetuses that do not grow properly have a higher mortality rate, usually show a variety of problems in the perinatal period and are at

Table 2 Prenatal growth profile. Variables and sonographic parameters

Variables	Measured parameters
Head size	head circumference (HC)
Trunk size	abdominal circumference (AC)
Soft tissue mass	thigh circumference
Length	femur length (FL)
Weight	estimated weight
Body proportionality	HC/AC, FL/HC ratios

high risk for long-term neurological problems. The clinical methods of assessing fetal size and growth – maternal weight gain, fundal height, abdominal circumference – are relatively imprecise, whereas the measurements of an image of the fetus obtained by ultrasound have been demonstrated to have a better capacity to detect abnormalities in fetal growth[9].

Changes in anatomic parameters are the most used indicators of the fetal growth process:

(1) Three-dimensional parameters, such as fetal weight and volume[10];

(2) Two-dimensional parameters, such as area of a profile of a body segment[11,12];

(3) One-dimensional parameters including either the diameter or the circumference of various body segments[13].

According to Deter and Harrist[14], as the principal aim of fetal growth studies is to try to predict the type of newborn resulting from a given pregnancy, it would seem obvious in prenatal studies to use parameters that are similar to those used to characterize newborns. From an extensive review of the pediatric literature they concluded that evaluation of head size, trunk size, soft tissue mass, weight, length and body proportions is required to obtain a good characterization of most growth problems. This group of variables was called the 'Prenatal growth profile' (Table 2).

The rationale for parameter selection is that these measurements should be well defined, easily measured, reliable and reasonably insensitive to technical error; moreover, prenatal and postnatal values should be compared directly.

We focus, for the most used parameters, on technical aspects and possible errors in measurements, deriving the data from a review of the literature.

Head size

A series of scans should be performed to find the long axis of the fetus. The probe should then be rotated through 90° to this axis, and angled so that the beam is along a transverse plane through the fetal head[15]. A series of parallel sections should be obtained in order to identify the following landmarks:

(1) Short midline;

(2) Cavum septum pellucidum;

(3) Thalami;

(4) Basal cisternae.

Inclusion of all four features means that the section includes both biparietal diameter (BPD) and occipitofrontal diameter (OFD) and can also be used to measure head circumference (HC) (Figure 3).

Having identified an appropriate section, measurements are made on a frozen image. For BPD, measurement is made from the leading edge of the echo from the proximal skull surface to the leading edge of the echo from the distal skull surface ('outer to outer'). Other authors use 'outer to inner', 'inner to

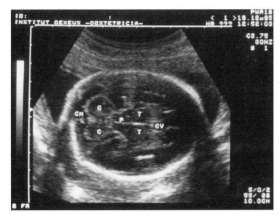

Figure 3 Section of the fetal head including the biparietal diameter (BPD) and the occipitofrontal diameter (the line perpendicular to the BPD). CV, cavum septum pellucidum; T, thalamus; C, cerebellum; CM, cisterna magna

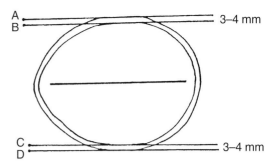

Figure 4 Line diagram showing several possibilities of positioning the electronic calipers to measure the biparietal diameter (BPD). If we measure from A (outer) to D (outer), the measurement will be 3–4 mm (or 3-4%) greater than that obtained by positioning one caliper in A (outer) and the other one in C (inner). Although the bone thickness of 3–4 mm is related to a third-trimester fetus, it represents 3–4% of the BPD also during the second trimester

outer' or 'middle to middle' measurement according to the positioning of electronic calipers with respect to the skull. It is important always to measure in the same fashion, comparing the results with curves obtained using the same method of measurement in order to avoid errors in over- or underestimations (up to 3–4% of obtained values) (Figure 4).

The OFD is obtained by positioning the calipers at both ends of the longest diameter perpendicular to the BDP. The HC measurement is made by tracing around the outer edge of the circumference of the image. Intra- and interobserver errors of –0.57% (± 2.1 SD) and 1.2% (± 4.4 SD), respectively, have been estimated[16]. At least two studies have shown that HC can be determined from BPD and OFD, assuming that the cross-section of the head in the BPD plane is an ellipse, with an accuracy similar to that obtained by direct measurement[17].

Head changes in shape, such as in dolicocephaly (BPD to OFD ratio < 0.75), affecting approximately 8% of fetuses, more frequently those in breech presentation, can affect single diameter measurement but they do not significantly affect the HC, which should be used in preference, at least in these cases. Moreover, prenatal and postnatal HC

values can be compared directly, since both measurements are made in the same location.

Trunk size

Among all the possible sections and parameters of the fetal trunk, the abdominal circumference (AC) has been chosen because it reflects changes in liver size which occur early in many fetuses with growth abnormalities (because of the availability and maintenance of blood glucose, for instance) and can be measured in a well-defined plane.

The long axis of the fetus is found by obtaining a longitudinal section through the fetal spine or aorta. The aorta is preferable to the spine, as it is not as wide as the spine, therefore minimizing the degree of obliquity of the true longitudinal plane. The transducer is then rotated through 90° to obtain a transverse image of the fetus at the level of the umbilical vein and of the stomach (Figure 5). The transverse section should be circular in outline as well as the outline of the aorta and the fetal spine[18]. These landmarks will be seen in several sections, but the correct one will show the portion of the umbilical vein situated most centrally as it enters the portal system within the liver. The umbilical vein

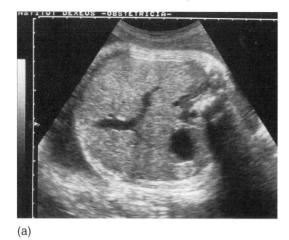

(a)

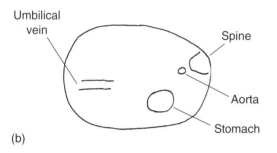

(b)

Figure 5 (a) Ultrasound image of appropriate section for the measurement of abdominal circumference. (b) Line diagram illustrating anatomical landmarks shown in (a)

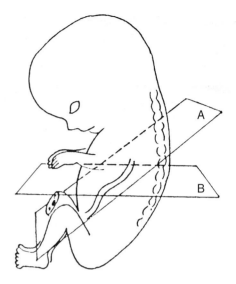

Figure 6 Representation of the umbilical vein course. A is the correct plane for the measurement of abdominal circumference; B is the incorrect plane

Comparison of pre- and postnatal AC measurements are affected by several variables, including the different levels of measurement and changes in liver position due to the initiation of breathing. Since these differences are systematic, they can be reduced by using an appropriate correction factor[20].

Length

The femur diaphysis length has been utilized as an indirect indicator of fetal length, since this parameter is strongly related with postnatal crown–heel length measurements[21].

The long axis of the fetus is found and the femora identified as the single long bones at its caudal end. The transducer is rotated until the longest possible image of the femur is obtained and the transducer is along the long axis of the femur (Figure 7). On the frozen image the femur image will have clear blunt ends, if the true long axis is obtained. A straight-line measurement is made between the two ends of the femoral diaphysis (the distal femoral epiphysis should not be included). The measurement is repeated until three values, all within 1 mm of each other,

runs in an anteroposterior and caudocranial direction, on a plane at approximately 40° to the longitudinal axis of the fetus (Figure 6). For this reason a cross-section of the fetal abdomen showing the umbilical vein from its insertion will be at approximately 50° to the correct plane and therefore unsuitable for measurements, which would be over-estimated.

When a satisfactory image is obtained, the circumference can be measured by tracing around the outer edge of the image. The intra- and interobserver errors have been reported to be –0.5% (±2.6 SD) and 2.4% (±1.6 SD), respectively[16]. As shown for HC, the AC values obtained from perpendicular diameters, assuming an elliptic shape for the cross-section of the fetal abdomen, are similar to those obtained by direct measurement[19].

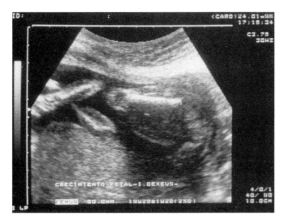

Figure 7 Femur length. The ultrasound image of the femur has clear sharp ends

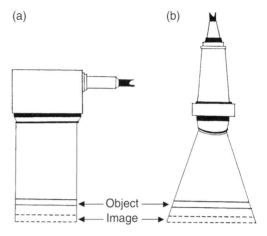

Figure 8 Effect of the difference in sound velocity on ultrasound measurements. By using a linear array probe (a) the apparent object is imaged 3.36% deeper than it actually is, but the apparent length is unaffected. By using a sector scanner (b) the apparent object is imaged 3.36% deeper than it actually is, but the apparent half-length is also increased by 3.36% through the rules of trigonometry

are obtained; the largest of these is considered as the femur length (FL)[18].

It should be noted that difference in orientation can affect this measurement, owing to the differences in axial and lateral resolution[22]. Consequently the femur should be measured when it is parallel or slightly oblique to the transducer.

Linear array scanners and sector scanners give different measurements of femur length, owing to the difference in apparent depth of the image (Figure 8). Although the difference is usually within acceptable limits (approximately 4%), the importance of these variations should be remembered when fetal age or growth is assessed during the third trimester[23].

Fetal weight

There are several situations (preterm labor, breech presentation, diabetes, previous Cesarean section) when it is of clinical value to have a single estimate of the fetal weight at one point in time. Formulae for using various ultrasonic parameters for estimating fetal weight are numerous, although no procedure is free of problems and errors as high as 15% can be expected with even the best methods. All the formulae tend to overstimate the weight of the low-weight fetus (< 1550 g) and understimate the weight of the high-weight fetus (> 4000 g)[24].

According to Deter and Harrist[14], although several methods appear to give similar results, those involving HC, AC and FL seem to be the most appropriate and consistent, since three of the five major body components (brain, trunk, skeleton, muscle and fat) are represented with minimal effects due to shape changes. They recommend the weight estimation function of Hadlock and co-workers[25]:

$$\log_{10} \text{weight} = 1.326 + 0.107(\text{HC}) + 0.0438(\text{AC}) + 0.158(\text{FL}) - 0.00326(\text{AC} \times \text{FL})$$

Body proportion

Several ratios of fetal anatomic parameters have been used for evaluation of body proportions. From a general point of view, ratios of head circumference to other body parts gradually decrease with increasing gestational age, while ratios not involving the head remain relatively constant after 20 weeks of gestation. The most popular are as follows.

The HC/AC ratio is commonly used to differentiate symmetric versus asymmetric growth anomalies, although this ratio has been proved to change considerably from one fetus to another in advancing gestational age[26].

The thoracic circumference (TC)/AC ratio is used in detecting pulmonary hypoplasia, although more recently Doppler studies have demonstrated a higher sensitivity[27].

The BPD/FL ratio has been used in screening for Down syndrome, usually in combination with other sonographic markers of chromosomal aberration[28].

The FL/HC ratio seems to be quite sensitive to both head (microcephaly) and long bone (dwarfism) growth abnormalities, although some skeletal dysplasia not involving head size and/or femur length may require measurement of other parameters[13].

References

1. Mahadevan N, Pearce M, Steer PH. The proper measure of intrauterine growth retardation is function, not size. *Br J Obstet Gynaecol* 1994;110:1032–5
2. Robinson HP. Sonar measurement of fetal crown–rump length as means of assessing maturity in first trimester of pregnancy. *Br Med J* 1973;4:28–31
3. Nelson LH. Comparison of methods for determining crown–rump measurement by real-time ultrasound. *J Clin Ultrasound* 1981;9:67–70
4. Drumm JE, Clinch J, Mackenzie G. The ultrasonic measurement of fetal crown–rump length as a method of assessing gestational age. *Br J Obstet Gynaecol* 1976;83:417–21
5. Hadlock FP, Shah YP, Kanon DJ, Lindsay JV. Fetal crown–rump length: reevaluation of relation to menstrual age (5–18 weeks) with high-resolution real time US. *Radiology* 1992;182:501–5
6. Selbing A, McKay K. Ultrasound in first trimester shows no difference in fetal size between the sexes. *Br Med J* 1985;290:750
7. Dubowitz LMS, Goldberg C. Assessment of gestation by ultrasound in various stages of pregnancy in infants differing in size and ethnic origin. *Br J Obstet Gynaecol* 1981;88:255–9
8. Pedersen JF. Ultrasound evidence of sexual difference in fetal size in first trimester. *Br Med J* 1980;281:1253
9. Altman DG, Hytten FE. Assessment of fetal size and fetal growth. In Chalmers Y, Enkin M, Kerse MJNC, eds. *Effective Care in Pregnancy and Childbirth*. Oxford: Oxford University Press, 1990: 411–18
10. Deter RL, Harrist RB, Hadlock FP, *et al.* Longitudinal studies of fetal growth using volume parameters determined with ultrasound. *J Clin Ultrasound* 1984;12:313
11. Cook LF, Cook PN. Volume and surface area estimators. *Automedica* 1981;4:13
12. Deter RL. Evaluation of studies of normal growth. In Deter RL, ed. *Quantitative Obstetrical Ultrasonography*. New York: Churchill Livingstone, 1986:65–112
13. Romero R, Pilu GL, Jeanty Ph, *et al. Prenatal Diagnosis of Congenital Anomalies*. Norwalk, CT: Appleton & Lange, 1988
14. Deter RL, Harrist BH. Assessment of normal fetal growth. In Chevernak F, Isaacson G, Campbell S, eds. *Ultrasound in Obstetrics and Gynecology*, Vol. 1. Boston: Little Brown, 1993:361–85
15. Hadlock FP, Deter RL, Harrist RB, *et al.* Fetal biparietal diameter: rational choice of plane of section for sonographic measurement. *Am J Roentgenol* 1982;138:871–4
16. Deter RL, Harrist RB, Hadlock FP, *et al.* Fetal head and abdominal circumferences. 1. Evaluation of measurement errors. *J Clin Ultrasound* 1982;10:357–63
17. Shields JR, Medearis AL, Bear MB. Fetal head and abdominal circumferences: ellipse calculations versus planimetry. *J Clin Ultrasound* 1987;15:237–9
18. British Medical Ultrasound Society. *Fetal Measurement Working Party Report. Clinical Applications of Ultrasonic Fetal Measurements*. London: British Institute of Radiology, 1990
19. Hadlock FP, Kent WR, Loyd JL, *et al.* An evaluation of two methods of measuring fetal head and body circumferences. *J Ultrasound Med* 1982;1:359–60
20. Deter RL, Hill RM, Tennyson LM. Predicting the birth characteristics of normal fetuses 14 weeks before delivery. *J Clin Ultrasound* 1989;17:89–93
21. Vintzileos AM, Campbell WA, Keckles S, *et al.* The ultrasound femur length as a prediction of fetal length. *Obstet Gynecol* 1984;64:779–82
22. Pretorius DH, Nelson FR, Manco-Johnson ML. Fetal age estimation by ultrasound: the impact of measurement errors. *Radiology* 1984;152:763
23. Jeanty P, Beck GJ, Chervenak FA, *et al.* A comparison of sector and linear array scanners for the measurement of the fetal femur. *J Ultrasound Med* 1985;4:525
24. Miller JM, Kissing GA, Brown HL, *et al.* Estimated fetal weight: applicability to small- and large-for-

gestational-age fetus. *J Clin Ultrasound* 1988;16: 95–7

25. Hadlock FP, Harrist RB, Sharman RS, *et al.* Estimation of fetal weight with the use of the head, body and femur measurements. A prospective study. *Am J Obstet Gynecol* 1985;151: 333–7

26. Deter RL, Harrist RB, Hadlock FP, *et al.* The ultrasound in assessment of normal fetal growth. *J Clin Ultrasound* 1981;9:481–93

27. Johnson A, Callan NA, Bhutani VK, *et al.* Ultrasonic ratio of fetal thoracic to abdominal circumference: an association with fetal pulmonary hypoplasia. *Am J Obstet Gynecol* 1987;157:764–9

28. Brumfields CG, Hauth JC, Cloud GA, *et al.* Sonographic measure-ments and ratios in fetuses with Down syndrome. *Obstet Gynecol* 1989;73:644–6

Definitions, etiology and clinical implications

3

J. M. Carrera

INTRODUCTION

Fetuses with intrauterine growth restriction (IUGR) greatly contribute to perinatal mortality and morbidity. IUGR undoubtedly constitutes one of the most challenging areas of research for obstetricians today. With other obstetric problems of concern having been solved, or well on the way to being solved, finding a solution to the problem of nutrient supply deficiency would appear to be our next goal if we are to continue to reduce, slowly but inexorably, the rate of perinatal mortality and the risk of mental and psychomotor retardation.

Despite marked progress made over the past decade in both diagnostic procedures and management strategies, the question of what causes growth restriction in 40% of all cases of IUGR still remains unanswered. On the other hand, IUGR continues to be associated with a three-fold to ten-fold increase in perinatal mortality; an increase in early perinatal morbidity due to congenital abnormalities, perinatal asphyxia and other neonatal processes (persistent fetal blood flow, hypothermia, hypoglycemia, polycythemia, etc.); and an increase in long-term morbidity (learning problems, abnormal behavior patterns, neurological deficits, etc.)[1-4].

DEFINITIONS

A clear distinction should be made between the meaning of three different terms – low birth weight, small for dates and IUGR – that tend to be considered to be synonymous.

Low birth weight

This term refers only to newborn infants weighing less than 2500 g independently of gestational age[5]. A distinction is made between low birth weight in newborns delivered before 37 weeks (preterm), low birth weight in newborns delivered between 37 and 42 weeks (full term) and low birth weight in newborns delivered after 42 weeks (post-term). Low birth weight may also be subdivided into 'very low birth weight' (1000 to 1499 g) and 'extremely low birth weight' (500 to 999 g).

Some of these newborns will be premature, and others will be newborns with IUGR. Accordingly, it is clear that 'fetal prematurity' and 'low birth weight in a fetus' are not terms that are synonymous, in the same manner that 'maturity', 'gestational age' and 'low birth weight' are not synonymous.

The expression 'premature newborn' implies a lack of maturity of the newborn to face extrauterine life and requiring special care to survive. It involves a biological concept that is impossible to define by any single measurement. Only with the help of a number of parameters will the neonatologist be able to assess whether the fetus will survive.

With regard to the term 'preterm newborn' the World Health Organization (WHO) in 1969 recognized the term to define all newborns with a gestational age of less than 37 weeks. The European Society of Perinatology (1971) and the FIGO (1975) used the same definition.

Small for gestational age (SGA)

This term is based on a statistical definition that includes all newborn infants found below the lower confidence limit of a normal weight–weeks of gestation curve. Depending upon the type of curve, the lower confidence limit may be the 3rd, 5th or 10th centile, or –1 or –2 SD.

In 1963, Gruenwald[6] proposed that growth-retarded newborns were those whose weight was 1 SD (probable or likely growth retardation) or 2 SD (growth retardation) below the mean weight for their age. In the same year, basing their calculations on a growth curve using the centile system, Lubchenco and colleagues[7] considered newborns below the 25th centile as small for gestational age or small-for-dates, although some years later they agreed to this definition for newborn infants below the 10th centile. Newborn infants between the 10th and the 90th centiles, however, were considered to be appropriate for gestational age and those over the 90th centile, large for gestational age. In 1966, Gruenwald[8] proposed using the 5th centile as an alternative limit, admitting that his first criterion of –2 SD was too strict.

Intrauterine growth restriction (IUGR)

IUGR refers to any process that is capable of limiting intrinsic fetal growth potential *in utero*. It is thus a heterogeneous entity with a variety of possible etiologies.

The term 'intrauterine growth retardation' was introduced by Warkani and co-workers[9] in 1961. The first obstetrician who stated that weight and age were not necessarily related was in fact Pierre Budin[10], in 1907, although it was not until 1947 that McBurney[11] provided proof of intrauterine growth retardation.

The distinction between IUGR and small for gestational age is important, since: first, some newborn infants may be termed small for gestational age (below the 5th or 10th centile) without having suffered IUGR; in this case, there are normal genetic reasons for their low birth weight (constitutional); and second, many cases of IUGR are not considered to be small for gestational age at birth. This is the case in fetuses that, given their high intrinsic growth potential, should weigh, for example, 4 kg at term but, as a result of an unfavorable gestational environment, weigh only 3 kg. In this case, they have suffered from IUGR but are considered to be 'appropriate for their gestational age'.

An evaluation of the postnatal ponderal index may help to establish which fetuses really have suffered deficiencies in intrauterine nutrient supply, independently of their weight at birth. Apparently, and in agreement with this index, 40% of fetuses termed small for gestational age should not be considered as suffering from IUGR[12].

Unfortunately, in the literature, the terms IUGR and SGA are frequently considered as synonymous. This confusion in terminology was increased even more when the National Institute of Child Health and Human Development in the USA[12] stated that for 'both medical and research purposes, intrauterine growth retardation should be defined as a situation which results in a newborn weight that is lower than the 10th percentile for its gestational age'.

INCIDENCE

The incidence of IUGR varies greatly in the literature, with reports of figures ranging from 1.1% to 10.8%[13]. The reason for this may be found in different factors, including:

(1) The definitions of birth weight, such as low birth weight, growth retardation with respect to gestational age, mixed categories;

(2) Different ways in which standard curves are drawn (centiles, standard deviations), data obtained from transverse or longitudinal studies, etc.[14];

(3) Different criteria used for discrimination (10th centile, 5th centile, –1 SD, –2 SD);

(4) The procedure by which the gestational age is calculated. Given the frequency of menstrual irregularity, especially in underdeveloped countries, if gestational age is calculated only from the last menstrual period (LMP), the incidence of IUGR can reach 20%. In contrast, if the gestational age is calculated from

biometric parameters, the incidence of true IUGR falls to 5%[15];

(5) Different geopolitical situations (while some northern countries have a very low rate of IUGR, some underdeveloped countries have very high rates; the factors influencing standard values in each country vary: height above sea level, degree of development of the country, ethnic characteristics) and social and economic status of the population under study in each country.

It is therefore difficult to compare the figures obtained in environments and countries that are very different, even when similar yardsticks are used. It is for this reason that each community (country, region, etc.) is encouraged to develop its own standard curve.

In our environment, the 10th centile has generally been accepted as the distinguishing criterion. If suitable, up-to-date curves were used for each community studied, the incidence of IUGR would, obviously, be 10%. However, this hardly ever occurs and figures reported usually range between 3% and 7%[16,17]. For obvious reasons, it is easier to compare figures obtained for 'low weight at birth'. In Spain, during the 10-year period between 1980 and 1989, the figure obtained was 5.7%[18], which is similar to 5.57% found in Catalonia in 1991.

According to gestational age, the majority of cases of IUGR occur at term, during weeks 38 to 42, followed by post-term and preterm pregnancies. The last account for only 1% of all neonates (Figure 1).

Gruenwald[6,8] emphasized the fact that almost one-third of newborns that weigh less than 2500 g are not premature, but newborns that are small for gestational age (SGA). Lugo and Cassady[19] elevated this figure to 44.9%.

ETIOLOGY

Innumerable factors are supposedly associated with variations in fetal birth weight. In the multicenter study carried out by Niswander and Gordon[20], 32 associated factors

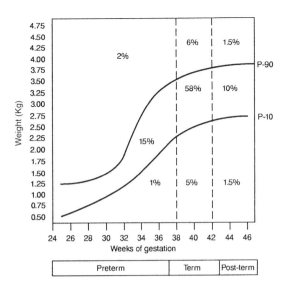

Figure 1 Incidence of intrauterine growth restriction according to gestational age

were identified and it is clear from an overall review of the literature that many more may be recognized. The etiological factors usually associated with IUGR may be divided into three groups: maternal factors, fetal factors and uteroplacental factors.

Maternal factors

This group includes the largest number of variables. The most common are as follows.

Constitutional factors

Maternal height It has been reported that for each centimeter by which maternal height exceeds normal values, fetal weight at birth is increased by 16 g[21]. When the weight factor is corrected, however, maternal height has little influence on the weight of the fetus[22].

Some investigators, such as Abdul-Karim and Beydoum[23], even believe that paternal weight is a more important factor than maternal weight in determining fetal weight. Recently, Wilcox and colleagues[24], in studying the relationship between fetal and paternal weights (multiple regression analysis, adjusting for mothers of normal size), concluded that if the father is of low stature (2 SD below the mean), the newborn will weigh, on average, 183 g less than if the father is of greater stature (2 SD above the mean).

Maternal weight at birth Ounsted and Ounsted[25] found a significant relationship between neonatal birth weight and maternal birth weight and suggested a strong hereditary influence on fetal variables.

Maternal weight prior to pregnancy Simpson and associates[26] have shown a clear correlation between maternal and fetal weights. Fetal growth retardation is particularly associated with mothers weighing less than 54 kg.

Maternal age The incidence of neonates with low weight at birth in women under the age of 20 is double that in women between the ages of 25 and 30. There is also a greater relative risk of fetal malnutrition (vascular and metabolic disorders, and a larger number of fetal chromosomal abnormalities) in older women[27-31].

Social and economic status

Unfavorable socioeconomic conditions clearly increase the incidence of neonates with low weight at birth. This is particularly true in developing countries. Factors include diet, social and family environment, education, type of work, teenage pregnancies or marital status, among others.

It is important to keep in mind that the most important factor in this regard is the poor nutrition or malnutrition of the mother. In this context, one of the most conclusive examples in the literature is the study by Gruenwald[32-34], who compared the weight of Japanese newborns in two distinct time periods. While Japanese newborn weights varied significantly from their American counterparts during a period of severe nutritional deprivation (1945–46), this difference was barely noticeable when nutrition in Japan had returned to normal (Figure 2).

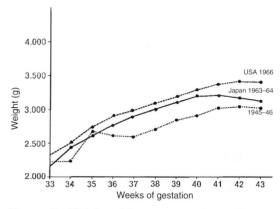

Figure 2 Weight of Japanese newborns in two distinct time periods (1945–46: severe nutritional deprivation; and 1963–64: normal period), compared with American counterparts

The effects of maternal malnutrition in development and in perinatal mortality in developing countries has been well studied by Lechtig and co-workers[35-37]. The statistics shown by these authors demonstrate significant differences in the percentage of low-birth-weight newborns in communities that are well nourished (in this case, a white urban population in the USA) and other communities with unfavorable socioeconomic conditions, both urban and rural. In these same geographic areas, higher-class populations had the same percentage of low-birth-weight newborns as in the control group, thus eliminating other possible variable factors such as race, geographic area, mean temperature, etc. To confirm their conclusions, Lechtig and colleagues compared three different socioeconomic classes in Guatemala, observing some very significant differences.

Lechtig and associates[37] elaborated a high-risk indicator for nutritional deficit that takes into account maternal height, cephalic circumference and household characteristics. It serves to increase the efficacy of aid programs in countries with limited resources.

A similar study by Norska[38] in Poland observed significant differences in the socioeconomic conditions of mothers who give birth to newborns with IUGR, as compared to a control group. For example, while the percentage of single mothers in the control group was 1.2%, it increased to 6.9% in the group with IUGR newborns. Drillien[39] observed that the incidence of premature and IUGR newborns bore a greater relationship to the socioeconomic status of the maternal grandfather than to that of the paternal grandfather, suggesting a possible influence of maternal nutritional history and state of health during her infancy.

Probably the greatest demonstration of the importance of maternal nutrition is obtained by observing that by supplementing the diet (extra protein, etc.) the incidence of newborns with low birth weight is reduced in a given community. In gravid women who have a caloric and protein deficit in their diet, an adequate supplement greatly diminishes the incidence of newborns with low birth weight.

It is clear that, by improving services and nutrition in a given community, there is an improvement in the mortality and nutrition of newborns[40]. Lechtig has even demonstrated a correlation between diverse categories of caloric supplements administered from conception and the incidence of IUGR.

Murthy and co-workers[41] studied the relationship between, on the one hand, daily ingestion of calories and proteins in different communities with normal or poor nutrition and, on the other hand, fetal weight and placental biometry (weight, volume, surface, number of cotyledons), by constructing the respective linear regressions. They observed an excellent correlation, especially between caloric intake and fetal and placental weight, and between protein intake and placental volume.

One of the parameters that may serve as a possible indicator of malnutrition of the fetus is poor maternal weight gain during pregnancy. There are various reports that support this[42,43]. Ademowore and associates[44] correlated maternal weight gain not only with fetal weight, but also with selected socioeconomic factors (income, race, etc.), confirming these relationships. Other authors

such as Hediger and colleagues[45] considered poor maternal weight gain by 12 weeks of gestation (less than the 10th centile) to be predictive of poor maternal weight gain later in pregnancy. One should be alert to the risk of IUGR in patients who fail to gain 3 kg by 20 weeks of gestation, or less than 1 kg per month thereafter[46].

Geographic and climatic factors

On occasion, it is difficult to separate geographic factors from socioeconomic factors (areas of endemic poverty), but the repercussions of the temperature and altitude of a given country on newborn weight seem evident.

Altitude above sea level Chronic maternal hypoxia conditioned by living at greater altitudes may play a role in limiting fetal and placental growth[47]. According to the statistics of Lichty and colleagues[48], in the county of Lake Colorado (10 000 feet above sea level) the average newborn weight was 3.07 kg, whereas in Denver (5000 feet above sea level) the average weight at birth was 3.29 kg and in Baltimore (at sea level) it increased to 3.32 kg. This report can be considered quite objective if one assumes that racial and nutritional factors in the three studied communities were similar.

Climatic conditions Some authors believe that there is a correlation between the average fetal weight and the mean annual temperature of a given area. Nevertheless, it is difficult to evaluate this correlation because of multiple confounding variables (race, socioeconomic conditions, etc.). Toverud[49] contends that the birth weight of babies born in the summer is significantly greater than that of babies born in the winter. He attributes this difference not to winter starvation, but to differences in the production of energy and the regeneration of maternal tissues stimulated by the cold and inactivity.

In contrast, Prasaad[50] reported that, in India, newborn birth weight was systematically lower during the summer and rainy months than during the winter. He also suggested that there is a slight increase in the incidence of IUGR in winters that follow hot summers compared to winters that follow cooler summers.

Race It is very difficult to find studies evaluating women of different ethnic groups that are strictly controlled for other variables such as socioeconomic status. It is difficult to separate genetic factors from other factors relating to nutritional status, socioeconomic class and environmental factors.

As Gruenwald[32] stated, it is difficult to appreciate to what degree purely racial factors contribute to fetal weight until diverse ethnic groups have lived under similar circumstances and environmental factors for a given time period, perhaps for two generations.

Nevertheless, there is a copious amount of information available that demonstates some ethnic differences that seem quite evident. Even if one accounts for socioeconomic and environmental differences, it appears evident that there are differences in newborn weight in white and black populations that are attributable, in at least half the cases, to purely racial influences[51]. According to Hendricks[46], a fetus of white race weighs 156 g more than the average weight of a fetus of black race at 40 weeks of gestation. In addition, the placenta, in the first case, weighs approximately 20 g more than in the black fetus. The difference, thus, is 4.8% for the fetus and 3.3% for the placenta. Aware of the possibility of confounding factors such as socioeconomic status and parity, Hendricks made the appropriate corrections in his data and arrived at the same conclusions.

A good example of the possible role of ethnicity in birth weight is demonstrated by Jans[52], who observed that the Bambuti pygmies in the tropical rain forests of the Itui have a very low average birth weight (2.635 kg), with an extraordinarily small variation (SD 0.332) compared to the usual findings in Caucasian newborns.

Toxic habits Smoking, alcohol use and drug consumption are included in this group. Different studies have demonstrated that, after excluding other variables, the weight at birth is reduced by an average of 170–200 g in infants born to mothers who smoke more than ten cigarettes a day[5,53–55].

Ulleland[56], in 1972, reported for the first time that IUGR was particularly common among children born to alcoholic mothers. Subsequently, other authors[57–59] described the characteristics of these children and established the concept of fetal alcoholic syndrome, in which weight, size and head circumference of neonates are found below the 3rd centile.

Finally, babies born to heroin-addicted mothers weigh significantly less than those born to mothers who do not consume opioids[60], independently of maternal nutrition during pregnancy.

Maternal diseases

Chronic renal disease Chronic renal diseases most frequently associated with IUGR include chronic pyelonephritis, glomerulosclerosis, chronic glomerular disease and lupus nephritis[61–63].

Chronic hypertension This is one of the most frequent causes of IUGR. It usually affects multiparas and gives rise to early growth retardation and microsomic neonates with learning and psychomotor problems.

Pre-eclampsia In studying important series of pre-eclamptics, a statistically significant reduction in fetal weight is noted, not only because of the higher incidence of prematurity in these patients, but also because of true IUGR[64]. These facts correlate well with our own experience.

For a long time it was believed that uteroplacental ischemia constituted the most important factor in fetal distress and hypotrophy in these cases. Vascular spasms would explain the majority of cases of sudden intrauterine fetal demise. In fact, it seems indisputable that in the course of the pregnancies of toxemic patients, blood flow to the uterus is greatly diminished and therefore results in fetal hypotrophy. It seems equally well confirmed that, in cases of toxemic patients and fetal hypotrophy, oxygen consumption by the placenta is diminished.

In recent years, a new theory has been proposed of some coagulation imbalance that links both of these processes. This hypothesis is supported by the observation of inter- and perivillus fibrin deposits, in addition to multiple infarcts in the placentas of some small-for-dates newborns delivered to toxemic mothers.

Finally, it is now widely accepted that there exists a pathological increase in the thromboxin/prostacyclin ratio, first at the level of the intervillus space and also at the level of the systemic circulation secondary to a deficiency in the production of prostacyclins of trophoblastic origin[65]. This imbalance in the thromboxin/prostacyclin ratio leads to an increase in systemic resistance and vasopressor sensitivity with a reduction in plasma volume. Additionally, there is an activation of coagulation, with an increase in platelet aggregation and thrombocytopenia, and of the vaso-constrictive phenomenon, both at the local and the systemic level (causing vasospasm and hypertension), all of which lead to reduced systemic perfusion and to a reduction in uteroplacental blood flow, with consequent IUGR[66–68].

This imbalance, according to O'Brien and Pipkin[69], clearly alters vascular sensitivity to angiotensin II. Nevertheless Kingdom and colleagues[70] have shown the activation of the fetal renin–angiotensin axis in IUGR, suggesting a normal sensitivity of the fetoplacental vasculature to this peptide, in spite of elevated levels of angiotensin II in the plasma. They suggest that this might cause an increase in the vascular resistance of the placenta.

Chronic cardiopulmonary disease IUGR has been reported in patients with heart or lung disease causing hypoxemia, such as congenital cardiopathies, coarctation of the aorta,

pulmonary atresia and reduced cardiac output, and pulmonary diseases, such as bronchial asthma and bronchiectasis.

Dysglycemias Long-standing, poorly controlled insulin-dependent diabetes associated with diabetic retinopathy, hypertension and nephritis may cause placental microvascular disorders that give rise to an increase in IUGR. In pregnancy-induced diabetes, a marked decrease in fetal weight may be due to excessive caloric reduction.

Autoimmune diseases The association between systemic lupus erythematosus and IUGR is well known, although it is usually difficult to distinguish between the effects of high doses of glucocorticoids and azathioprine, and vasculitis caused by the disease[71]. On the other hand, antiphospholipid syndrome (lupus-like) has been associated with an increase in the number of cases of miscarriage, IUGR and intrauterine deaths[72–75].

Anemia Whilst low levels of hemoglobin (less than 6 g/dl) are associated with an increase in perinatal mortality, moderate anemia (6–10 g/dl) is associated with a significant decrease in fetal weight[76,77]. This may be due to a decrease in oxygen transport (as in sickle cell anemia) or it may simply be related to poor maternal nutrition.

Urinary tract infection It has been generally accepted that pyelonephritis during pregnancy causes IUGR[61].

Fetal factors

Fetal gender In accordance with data collected from various sources[46,78,79], the male fetus at term weighs on average 140–150 g more than his female counterpart. The difference is 4%. As a consequence, if sex-adjusted curves are not used, the incidence of IUGR is greater in female fetuses.

Chromosome abnormalities Chromosome abnormalities, in particular trisomies 13, 18 and 21, as well as Turner syndrome (45,X), sex chromosomal trisomy (XXX, XYY, XXY) or segmental chromosome imbalances (4p – short arm, 5p – cri-du-chat syndrome, 18p, 18q, etc.) are accompanied by a high incidence of IUGR, which occurs early in pregnancy (IUGR type I). It is for this reason that antenatal ultrasonographic diagnosis of growth retardation of this type should be followed by a study of fetal karyotype using the most appropriate method in each case (amniocentesis, chorionic villus biopsy or cordocentesis).

Inherited syndromes A variety of diseases of bone and cartilage have been called dysplasias, e.g. dwarfism (achondroplasia, hypo-chondroplasia, Russell–Silver syndrome), chondrodystrophies, osteogenesis imperfecta, etc. Placental sulfatase deficiency has also been cited as causing IUGR.

Fetal infection As a result of the epidemic of rubella in 1963, it was established that transplacental infection of the fetus can cause IUGR. Since 1963, numerous reports have appeared, associating low fetal weight with intrauterine infections such as rubella, cytomegalovirus, herpes simplex, toxo-plasmosis, paludism, congenital syphilis and other acute bacterial infections. Unfortunately, most reports make no distinction between premature and small-for-dates neonates.

Twin pregnancies This is one of the most frequent and well-known causes of IUGR. In all series of IUGR, twin pregnancies account for 20–30% of the cases. The intrauterine growth curve of twin pregnancies is similar to that of singleton pregnancies until week 33 of gestation; from then on, the curve for monozygotic twins diverges; that of dizygotic twins does so between weeks 35 and 36.

Immunological factors In animal studies, the 'dwarf syndrome', has been described in which there is a severe limitation of growth in newborns when there is an exacerbation of host-versus-fetal graft syndrome.

In humans, in some cases, immunological factors play an important role in the development of certain types of IUGR. Some examples which demonstrate this are the limitation of fetal weight in some fetuses that have undergone intrauterine transfusions; the increase in genetic alterations in pregnancies complicated by incompatibility of the human leukocyte antigen (HLA); and the similarity between certain placental histological alterations in fetuses with IUGR and those found in animals with the 'dwarf syndrome'[80].

Fetal order at birth IUGR occurs more often in first-born neonates, particularly when the mother is very young or of advanced age. The second or third child of the same mother usually weighs more than the first child. What happens as from the fourth child on is not clear, as the series studied are small. In most countries, women who have more than three children frequently belong to the lower social classes. This may be a factor in decreased fetal weight.

Uteroplacental factors

Uterine anomalies Congenital uterine anomalies, in particular uterus bicornis and septate uterus, are consistently associated with IUGR, and account for approximately 1–3% of the cases.

Poor adaptation of maternal circulation There is growing evidence that poor circulation prior to pregnancy, with or without deficiencies in uterine vasculature, can give rise to repeated miscarriages and very early growth retardation[81]. Inadequate vascular supply, whether anatomical or functional, prevents correct placental implantation and circulatory anchorage. Color Doppler imaging is currently being used to study placental blood supply. It may well provide the key to the early diagnosis of pregnancies in which these conditions occur.

Poor adaptation of maternal circulation may also be associated with immunological factors[82,83]. This would seem to be particularly so in the case of early IUGR in the presence of antiphospholipid antibodies (lupus anticoagulant and anticardiolipin antibodies). In this case, the cause may lie in an early inhibition of the production of prostacyclin at the level of the vascular endothelium[84]. However, more specific immunological studies are required to determine the mechanism linking poor vascular support with immunological rejection, very early growth retardation and possible fetal death.

Placental mosaicism Numerous cases of placental aneuploidies have been described, particularly trisomies 2, 7, 9, 10, 12, 13, 15, 16 and 18, that have been associated with miscarriages, growth retardation and fetal death, despite the fact that fetuses were chromosomally normal[84–90]. Kalousek and Dill[84] suggested that the occurrence of non-disjunction at random in the very early stages after conception could have given rise to mosaicism in the placenta or in the fetus, but not necessarily in both.

According to Kalousek and associates[86], three types of placental mosaicism may be defined:

(1) Type I, the most common, which may be found in cytotrophoblastic cells by carrying out a chorionic villus biopsy for karyotyping, by the direct method of Simoni. Fetal outcome is good.

(2) Type II, in which the abnormal karyotype is confined to mesenchymal cells. Diagnosis by chorionic villus biopsy can be made only with prolonged cell culture. It is not as common as type I and usually causes quite severe cases of IUGR.

(3) Type III, in which aneuploidy is present not only in the cytotrophoblast but also in mesenchymal cells. This occurs rarely, and it very often causes severe IUGR and fetal death.

There is a high correlation between the number of aneuploid cells detected by chorionic villus biopsy and the number confirmed in studies of the placenta at term. This also has its influence on fetal outcome. Growth retardation (80% of cases) and fetal death (20–30% of cases) normally need be feared only in cases of high levels of mosaicism (more than 45% of cells involved)[91–94]. For this reason it has been suggested[86], at least in part, that the length of gestation and fetal survival depend upon the ratio of euploid cells to aneuploid cells in the placenta. Many other conceptions are, however, aborted before 22 weeks' gestation. Nevertheless, there are case reports of normal fetuses[95,96].

PATHOGENESIS

Three mechanisms are currently recognized: decrease in intrinsic fetal growth potential, uteroplacental insufficiency and fetal malnutrition secondary to maternal malnutrition.

Decrease in intrinsic fetal growth potential

Different etiological factors, such as those of genetic and/or chromosomal origin, toxic habits or infectious diseases, cause a decrease in intrinsic fetal growth potential. The pathological noxa begin to exert their influence from the time of conception or, at least, from the embryonic stage.

In certain chromosome abnormalities, such as those involving sex chromosomes, particularly with an excess number of chromosomes in the karyotype, a progressive, linear decrease in fetal weight has been detected. Thus, for every extra X chromosome, fetal weight loss would be 300 g.

Embryopathic infectious processes may influence intrinsic fetal growth potential in several ways, either by first affecting the mother, thereby directly affecting the fetus, or by negatively affecting both. When they directly affect the fetus during the stages of organ differentiation, they are capable of causing a permanent reduction in the number of cells, thereby causing more or less severe damage to most of the fetal organs.

Rubella and cytomegalovirus infection are the most significant. Cytomegalovirus, in particular, would appear to be responsible for a large number of cases of IUGR that are often considered idiopathic.

Uteroplacental insufficiency

This includes all factors capable of affecting maternal–placental–fetal exchange, usually as a result of deficiencies in the placental microcirculation. Uteroplacental insufficiency usually occurs in the presence of unfavorable conditions (e.g. insertion anomalies of the placenta, uterine blood flow impairment (as well as determining factors (e.g. pre-eclampsia, hypertension prior to pregnancy, renal disease, diabetes, post-term pregnancy). None of these factors usually come into play unless the fetus requires the reserve capacity of the placenta.

The main pathological finding is a significant decrease in the number of arterioles in the tertiary villi[97], which may be the result of two basic pathogenetic mechanisms: first, no formation of arterioles due to interference in the process of placental maturation angiogenesis[98]; or second, obliteration, secondary to a thromboembolic or angiospastic phenomenon[99]. In both cases, the cause of these changes may ultimately lie in a decrease in uterine perfusion, or in the fetus itself.

Impaired uterine perfusion causes hypoxic ischemia in the intervillous space with secondary constriction of villus arterioles[100]. In this case, changes in uterine blood flow velocity waveforms may be detected in Doppler studies before changes are detected in umbilical velocity waveforms, as occurs, for example, in patients with pre-eclampsia[101,102].

Evidence currently exists of the fact that the fetus itself, through poorly understood reflex or biochemical mechanisms, may induce changes in villous microcirculatory resistance. This occurs, for example, in fetuses with certain chromosome or morphological anomalies[99,103–105].

The study of the placenta in fetuses with autosomal trisomy reveals decreased vasculature in tertiary villi[106], which accounts for the reduced umbilical conductance indices and frequent episodes of distress observed in this type of fetus.

Exactly how chromosome anomalies act on the placenta to cause these anomalies is still unknown. It has been suggested, in the case of trisomy 21 in particular, that these anomalies make the placenta more susceptible to disrupting environmental influences[103,105], a concept known as 'enhanced development of instability'[105]. It is, however, still not clear how this susceptibility is mediated at cellular or subcellular level, thereby causing deficient cell proliferation, changing the cell cycle or modifying cell DNA or rRNA content.

Other researchers[98,99] have shown that, in a statistically significant percentage of placentas from fetuses with certain abnormalities, there was a significant decrease in the number of arterioles in tertiary villi. The most commonly occurring malformations in this group were those affecting the central nervous system.

Current research is focused on identifying the teleological mechanism by which the embryo or fetus affects the placenta, thereby causing placental insufficiency. The fact is that under these circumstances, although the umbilical velocity waveforms may be affected, uteroplacental velocity waveforms remain unaffected[98,107–110].

Fetal malnutrition secondary to maternal malnutrition

The physiopathological cause of low fetal birth weight may be found in an unsuitable composition of maternal blood, which causes an almost constant nutritional and metabolic deficiency in the fetus throughout pregnancy. Etiological factors include maternal nutritional deficits, poor living conditions, anemia, severe placental dystrophy, maternal hyperinsulinism (pregnant women with baseline and post-prandial hypoglycemia) and poor weight gain as a result of an unbalanced diet.

CLASSIFICATION OF IUGR

The first classification of IUGR that was widely used was that proposed by Winick and colleagues[111–115]. On the basis of experimental studies in rats, two types of IUGR were proposed:

(1) 'Intrinsic', caused by a decrease in fetal growth potential;

(2) 'Extrinsic', caused by placental insufficiency (asymmetrical IUGR), or maternal protein restriction (symmetrical IUGR).

This classification was accepted, with only slight variations, by the majority of English-language authors[116,117], and has come to be taken for granted in most texts on the subject.

On the basis of sonographic features, Campbell and associates[118,119] proposed a classification of IUGR largely based on the profile of the fetal biparietal diameter curve. These authors distinguished between IUGR with an 'early low profile' in the cephalometric curve and IUGR with a downturn or 'late flattening' of the curve. This classification, adopted by most specialists in ultrasonography, was later added to by Levi and colleagues[120,121], who also took into account the head circumference/abdominal circumference (HC/AC) index. Following this classification, IUGR was divided into 'harmonious' or 'proportionate' (normal HC/AC ratio) and 'disharmonious' or 'disproportionate' (increased HC/AC ratio). Experience soon showed that cases of IUGR classified as harmonious were usually intrinsic and exhibited an early low cephalometric profile; by contrast, cases of IUGR classified as disharmonious were extrinsic and exhibited a late flattening of the cephalometric curve.

Most English-language authors[122] subsequently adopted the classification of symmetrical or asymmetrical IUGR, with some[123] adding a third category known as symmetrical IUGR with 'femur sparing', characterized by femur length appropriate for gestational age but out of proportion to all other biometric parameters.

From the point of view of the characteristics of the newborn infant (presence or absence of malformations, biometric data, trophism, etc.), several classifications have been proposed. Rosso and Winick[124] identified IUGR accompanied by congenital malformations, and IUGR without congenital malformations. The latter group is subdivided into type I (extrinsic symmetrical) and type II (extrinsic asymmetrical). In 1977, Sieroszewski[125] and Holtorff[126] each proposed their own, very similar, classifications. The former divided fetuses that were small for gestational age into hypoplastic and hypotrophic, and the second divided them into eutrophic (genetically small), hypoplastic, hypotrophic and with multiple congenital malformations.

In practice, most pediatric departments classify cases of IUGR as proportionate (or symmetrical) and disproportionate (or asymmetrical) by calculating the ponderal index of Rohrer (fetal weight divided by fetal length (crown–rump), raised to the third power and multiplied by 100). If the index is normal (≥ 2.20), IUGR is considered symmetrical; if it is abnormally low, IUGR is considered asymmetrical[127–131].

Soothill and associates[132], using ultrasound scanning techniques, identified three types of SGA: abnormal SGA (chromosomal, structural or infective abnormality); fetal growth restricted SGA (placental dysfunction with abnormal umbilical Doppler; and normal SGA (normal placental function). This last group simply represents one end of the normal-size spectrum.

Depending upon the severity of IUGR, it has been classified as slight, moderate or severe[133].

Integrated classification of IUGR

This classification has been proposed by our group[134–145] since 1976 and takes into account all the basic aspects of IUGR, such as onset (early or late), etiology (intrinsically abnormal developmental process, etc.), anthropometric data of the newborn infant (weight, length, head circumference), general morphology (proportionate, disproportionate, semi-proportionate) and trophism (eutrophic, hypotrophic, dystrophic). In accordance with these characteristics, three types of IUGR have been recognized (Table 1):

Table 1 Types of intrauterine growth restriction

	Type I	*Type II*	*Type III*
Abnormal anthropometric parameters	weight, size and heart perimeter	weight	weight and size
General morphology	harmonious	disharmonious	semiharmonious
Origin	intrinsic	extrinsic pathological	extrinsic (deficiency)
Starting point	early	late	semi-early
Trophism	hypoplastic eutrophic	dystrophic underfed	hypotrophic badly fed

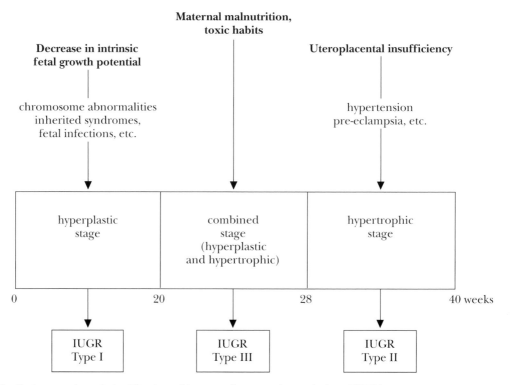

Figure 3 Pathogenesis and classification of intrauterine growth restriction (IUGR)

(1) Type I implies a decrease in intrinsic fetal growth potential and is also known as intrinsic, harmonious, proportionate, symmetrical or early. In this case, the noxa exert their influence from the time of conception, or at least from the embryonic stage (hyperplastic stage) (Figure 3). Owing to the early onset of the process, the three parameters that are usually assessed to determine IUGR are uniformly affected: fetal weight, length and head circumference. Newborn infants are hypoplastic or microsomic, but their appearance is clearly eutrophic. The incidence of congenital malformations is very high (aneuploidy in 25% of fetuses with severe growth restriction in the early stages of gestation)[146]. It is therefore advisable to carry out routine studies of the fetal karyotype. Approximately 20–30% of cases of IUGR are of this type[132,147,148].

(2) Type II, known as extrinsic, disharmonious, disproportionate, asymmetrical or late, in which uteroplacental insufficiency is the etiopathogenetic mechanism. Since factors involved in uteroplacental insufficiency are particularly common during the last trimester of pregnancy (hypertrophic stage), only fetal weight is affected whilst little or no effect is evident in fetal length or head circumference. The physical appearance of the neonate is characteristic, with a disproportionately large head and dystrophic, under-nourished body. Cases of *in utero* fetal death and fetal distress during delivery are most often found in this group. Approximately 70–80% of cases of IUGR are thought to be of this type[118].

(3) Type III, somewhat mixed in comparison with the other two types since, while the factors at work are apparently extrinsic and appear relatively early in pregnancy (nutrient deficiency), the consequences are more akin to those associated with intrinsic IUGR where fetal weight and length, in particular, are modified. Neonates in this group are characterized by semiharmonious morphology and a hypotrophic, undernourished appearance.

References

1. Butler NR, Alberman ED, eds. *Second Report of British Perinatal Mortality Survey. Perinatal Problems.* Edinburgh: Livingstone, 1969
2. Bard H. Intrauterine growth retardation. *Clin Obstet Gynecol* 1970;13:511–25
3. Teberg AJ, Walther FJ, Pena IC. Mortality, morbidity and outcome of the small-for-gestational age infants. *Semin Perinatol* 1988;12:84–94
4. Fabre E, González de Agüero R, De Agustín JL, Repollés S, Tajada M. Epidemiología del crecimiento intrauterino retardado: análisis de los datos de la Encuesta Nacional de Mortalidad Perinatal desde 1980 hasta 1989. *V Curso Internacional sobre 'Avances en gineco-obstetricia y reproducción humana'*, Barcelona, May 1992
5. World Health Organization. Aspects of low birth weight. Report of the Expert Committee of maternal child health. *WHO Technical Report* 1961; 217:3–16
6. Gruenwald P. Chronic fetal distress and placental insufficiency. *Biol Neonate* 1963;5:215–21
7. Lubchenko L, Hansman C, Dressler M, Boyd E. Intrauterine growth as estimated from liveborn birth weight data at 24 to 42 weeks of gestation. *Pediatrics* 1963;32:793–800
8. Gruenwald P. Growth of the human fetus. 1. Normal growth and its variation. *Am J Obstet Gynecol* 1966;94:1112–19
9. Warkani J, Monroe B, Ystherland BS. Intrauterine growth retardation. *Am J Dis Child* 1961;102:249–79
10. Budin P. *The Nursling. The Feeding and Hygiene of Premature and Full Term Infants.* Maloney WJ (transl.). London: Caxton Publishing, 1907
11. McBurney RD. The undernourished full term infant. *West J Surg Obstet Gynecol* 1947;55:363
12. Read MS, Catz C, Grave G, McNellis D, Warshaw JB. Introduction: intrauterine growth retardation – identification of research needs and goals. *Semin Perinatol* 1984;8:2–4
13. Branconi F, Faldi P, Mello G, *et al.* The poor endouterine growth of the fetus in treated diabetic patients. In Salvadori B, Bacchi-Modena A, eds. *Poor Intrauterine Fetal Growth.* Parma: Minerva Medica, 1977
14. Keirse MJNC. Aetiology of intrauterine growth retardation. In Van Assche A, Robertson WB, eds. *Fetal Growth Retardation.* Edinburgh: Churchill Livingstone, 1981:37–56
15. Grennert L, Persson P, Gennser G. Benefits of ultrasound screening of a pregnant population. *Acta Obstet Gynecol Scand* 1978;78(Suppl):5–14
16. Berkowitz RL, Hobbins JC. Ultrasonography in the antepartum patient. In Bolognese RJ, Schwartz R, eds. *Perinatal Medicine Management in the High Risk Fetus and Neonate.* Baltimore: Williams and Wilkins, 1977:85–112
17. Galbraith RS, Karchmar EJ, Pievey WN, *et al.* The clinical prediction of intrauterine growth retardation. *Am J Obstet Gynecol* 1979;133:281–6
18. CMBDAH. Análisi dels parts i variables perinatals. Any 1989. *Butll Epidemiol Catalunya* 1991;12:37–9
19. Lugo G, Cassady G. Intrauterine growth

retardation. Pathologic findings in 233 consecutive infants. *Am J Obstet Gynecol* 1971;109: 615–22

20. Niswander KR, Gordon M. *The Women and their Pregnancies.* Philadelphia: Saunders, 1972

21. Kloosterman GJ. On intrauterine growth: the significance of prenatal care. *Gynecol Obstet* 1970;8:895–904

22. Love EJ, Kinch RA. Factors influencing the birth weight in normal pregnancy. *Am J Obstet Gynecol* 1965;91:342–9

23. Abdul-Karim RW, Beydoum SN. Growth of the human fetus. *Clin Obstet Gynecol* 1974;17:37–52

24. Wilcox MA, Newton CS, Johnson IR. Paternal influences on birth weight. *Acta Obstet Gynecol Scand* 1995;74:15–18

25. Ounsted M, Ounsted C. Maternal regulation of intrauterine growth. *Nature (London)* 1968;87: 777–81

26. Simpson JW, Lawless RW, Cameron A. Responsibility of the obstetrician to the fetus: influence of pregnancy weight and pregnancy weight gain on birthweight. *Obstet Gynecol* 1975; 45:481–7

27. Hedberg E, Holmdahl K, Pehrson S. On relationship between maternal health and congenital malformations. *Acta Obstet Gynecol Scand* 1967;46:378

28. Papaevangelou G, Papadatos G, Alexiou D. The effect of maternal age, parity and social class on the incidence of small for dates newborns. *Acta Paediatr Scand* 1973;62:527–30

29. Hansen JP. Older maternal age and pregnancy outcome: a review of the literature. *Obstet Gynecol Surv* 1986;41:726–42

30. Grimes DA, Gross GK. Pregnancy outcomes in black women aged 35 and older. *Obstet Gynecol* 1981;58:614–20

31. Stein A. Pregnancy in gravidas over age 35 years. *J Nurse-Midwifery* 1983;28:17–20

32. Gruenwald P. Chronic fetal distress and placental insufficiency. *Biol Neonate* 1963;5:215–21

33. Gruenwald P. Growth of the human fetus. 1. Normal growth and its variation. *Am J Obstet Gynecol* 1966;94:1112–19

34. Gruenwald P. The relation of deprivation to perinatal pathology and late sequels. In Guenwald P, ed. *The Placenta.* Lancaster: Medical Technical Publishing, 1975

35. Lechtig A, Klein RE. Prenatal nutrition and birth weight: is there a causal association? In Dobbing JE, ed. *Maternal Nutrition in Pregnancy: Eating for Two?* London: Academic Press, 1981:131–56

36. Lechtig A, Habicht JP, Delgado H, Klein RE, Yarbrourgh C, Martorell R. Effect of food supplementation during pregnancy on birthweight. *Pediatrics* 1975;56:508–20

37. Lechtig A, Yarbrough C, Delgado H, Martorell

R, Klein RE, Behar M. Effect of moderate maternal malnutrition on the placenta. *Am J Obstet Gynecol* 1975;123:191–201

38. Norska J. Causes of intrauterine fetal dystrophy. In Salvadori B, Bacchi-Modena A, eds. *Poor Intrauterine Fetal Growth.* Parma: Minerva Medica, 1977:137–9

39. Drillien CM. The social and economic factors affecting the incidence of premature birth. 1. Premature births without complications of pregnancy. *Br J Obstet Gynaecol* 1957;64:161–84

40. Osofsky HJ. Relationship between nutrition during pregnancy and subsequent infant and child development. *Obstet Gynecol Surv* 1975;30: 227–41

41. Murthy LS, Agarwal DN, Khanna S. Placental morphometric and morphologic alterations in maternal undernutrition. *Am J Obstet Gynecol* 1976;124:641–6

42. Singer JE, Westphal M, Niswander K. Relationship of weight gain in pregnancy to birth weight and infant growth development in the first year of life. *Obstet Gynecol* 1968;31:417–23

43. Niswander KR, Singer J, Westphal M, Weiss W. Weight gain during pregnancy and prepregnancy weight: association with birth weight of term gestation. *Obstet Gynecol* 1969;33:482–91

44. Ademowore AS, Courey NG, Kime JJ. Relationship of maternal nutrition and weight gain to newborn birthweight. *Obstet Gynecol* 1972;39:460–4

45. Hediger ML, Scholl TO, Belsky DH, Ances IG, Salmon RW. Patterns of weight gain in adolescent pregnancy: effects on birth weight and preterm delivery. *Obstet Gynecol* 1989;74:6–12

46. Hendricks CH. Patterns of fetal and placental growth: the second half of normal pregnancy. *Obstet Gynecol* 1964;24:357–65

47. Krüger H, Arias-Stella J. The placenta and the newborn infant at high altitudes. *Am J Obstet Gynecol* 1970;106:586–91

48. Lichty JA, Ting RY, Buns PD, Dyar E. Studies of babies born at high altitude. Relation of altitude to birth weight. *AMAN Dis Child* 1957;93:666–78

49. Toverud KU. The vitamin C requirements of pregnant and lactating women. *Acta Pediatr* 1939; 24:332

50. Prasaad LS. Small for dates. *Indian J Pediatr* 1956; 23:115

51. Naylor AF, Myrianthopoulos NC. The relation of ethnic and selected socioeconomic factors to human birth weight. *Ann Hum Genet* 1967;31: 71–83

52. Jans, cited by Polani PE. Chromosomal and other genetic influences on birth weight

variations. In Elliot K, Knight, eds. *Size at Birth*. Amsterdam: Associated Scientific Publishers, 1974:127–64

53. Hasselmeyer ED, Meyer MB, Longo LD, *et al*. Pregnancy and infant health. In *The Health Consequences of Smoking Women. A Report of Surgeon General*. DHEW Publication 79-50069. Washington: Government Printing Office, 1980

54. Royal College of Physicians. *Smoking and Health Now*. London: Pitman, 1970

55. Hardy JB, Mellits DD. Does maternal smoking during pregnancy have a long-term effect on the child? *Lancet* 1973;2:1332–6

56. Ulleland CN. The offspring of alcoholic mothers. *Ann NY Acad Sci* 1972;197:167–9

57. Jones KL, Smith DW, Ulleland CN, Streissguth AP. Pattern of malformation in offspring of chronic alcoholic mothers. *Lancet* 1973;1:1267–71

58. Palmer RH, Oullette EM, Warner L, Leichtman SR. Congenital malformations in offspring of a chronic alcoholic mother. *Pediatrics* 1974;53:490–4

59. González-Merlo J, Mestres J, Urne J. Patrón de malformaciones en la descendencia de madres alcohólicas. Síndrome alcohólico fetal. Ponencia al Symposio sobre Subnormalidad Mental; Barcelona; 1977. In Esteban-Altirriba J, Sabater J, Balaña F, eds. *Prevención de la subnormalidad*. Barcelona: Salvat, 1979:313–44

60. Naeye RL, Blanc W, Leblanc W, Khatamee MA. Fetal complications of maternal heroin addiction: abnormal growth, infections and episodes of stress. *J Pediatr* 1973;83:1055–61

61. Katz AI, Davison JM, Hayslett JP, *et al*. Pregnancy in women with kidney disease. *Kidney Int* 1980;18:192–203

62. Surian M, Imbasciate E, Cosci P, *et al*. Glomerular disease and pregnancy: a study of 123 pregnancies in patients with primary and secondary glomerular disease. *Nephron* 1984;36:101–5

63. Jungers P, Forget D, Houllier P, Henry-Amar M, Grunfeld JP. Pregnancy in IgA nephropathy, reflux nephropathy and focal glomerular sclerosis. *Am J Kidney Dis* 1987;9:334–9

64. Zuspan FO. Adrenal gland and sympathetic nervous system response in eclampsia. *Am J Obstet Gynecol* 1972;114:304–13

65. Walsh SW. Thromboxane production in placentas of women with preeclampsia. *Am J Obstet Gynecol* 1989;160:1535–6

66. Remuzzi G, Marchesi D, Zoja C, *et al*. Reduced umbilical and placental vascular prostacyclin in severe preeclampsia. *Prostaglandins* 1980;20:105–10

67. Bussolino F, Benedetto C, Massobrio M, Camussi G. Maternal vascular prostacyclin activity in preeclampsia. *Lancet* 1980;2:702

68. Downing I, Sheperd GL, Lewis PJ. Reduced prostacyclin production in preeclampsia. *Lancet* 1980;2:1374

69. O'Brien PM, Pipkin FB. The effects of deprivation of prostaglandin precursors on vascular sensitivity to angiotensin II and on the kidney in the pregnant rabbit. *Br J Pharmacol* 1979;65:29–34

70. Kingdom JC, McQueen J, Cornell JMC, Whittle MJ. Fetal angiotensin II levels and vascular angiotensin receptors in pregnancies complicated by intrauterine growth retardation. *Br J Obstet Gynaecol* 1993;100:476–82

71. Fine LG, Barnett EV, Danowitch GM. Systemic lupus erythematosus in pregnancy. *Ann Intern Med* 1981;94:667–77

72. Lubbe WF, Liggins G. Lupus anticoagulant and pregnancy. *Am J Obstet Gynecol* 1985;153:322–7

73. Farquharson RC, Pearson JF, John L. Lupus anticoagulant and intrauterine death in the absence of systemic lupus. *Lancet* 1984;2:228–9

74. Branch DW, Scott JR, Kochenoor NK, Hershgold E. Obstetric complications associated with the lupus anticoagulant. *N Engl J Med* 1985;313:1322–6

75. Lockwood CJ, Romero R, Feinberg RF, Clyne LP, Coster B, Hoobins JC. The prevalence and biological significance of lupus anticoagulant and anticardiolipin antibodies in a general obstetric population. *Am J Obstet Gynecol* 1989;161:369–73

76. Beischer NA. The effects of maternal anemia upon the fetus. *J Reprod Med* 1971;6:262–3

77. Kuizon M, Cheong RL, Ancheta LP, Desnacido JA, Macapinlac MP, Baens JC. Effect of anemia and other maternal characteristics on birth weight. *Hum Nutr Clin Nutr* 1985;39C:419–26

78. Thompson AM, Billewitz WZ, Hytten FE. The assessment of fetal growth. *Br J Obstet Gynaecol* 1968;75:903–16

79. McKeown T, Record R. The influence of placental size of foetal growth in man, with special reference to multiple pregnancy. *J Endocrinol* 1953;9:418–26

80. Jones MD, Battaglia FC. Intrauterine growth retardation. *Am J Obstet Gynecol* 1977;127:540–9

81. Carrera JM, Mallafré J, Otero F, Rubio R, Carrera M. Síndrome de Mala Adaptación Circulatoria materna: Bases etiopatogénicas y terapéuticas. In Carrera JM, ed. *Doppler en Obstetricia*. Barcelona: Masson-Salvat, 1992:335–59

82. Mowbray JF, Underwood JC. Immunology of abortion. *Clin Exp Immunol* 1985;60:1–7

83. Scott JB, Rote NS, Branoh DW. Immunologic aspects of recurrent abortion and fetal death. *Obstet Gynecol* 1987;70:645–56

84. Kalousek DK, Dill FJ. Chromosomal mosaicism confined to the placenta in human conceptions. *Science* 1983;221:665–7

85. Kalousek DK, Dill FJ, Pantzar JJ, et al. Confined chorionic mosaicism in prenatal diagnosis. *Hum Genet* 1987;77:163–7

86. Kalousek DK, Barret I, McGuilliuray BC. Placental mosaicism and intrauterine survival for trisomies 13 and 18. *Am J Hum Genet* 1989;44:338–43

87. Kalousek DK, Howard-Peebles PN, Olson SB, et al. Confirmation of Cvs mosaicism in term placental and high frequency of intrauterine growth retardation association with confined placental mosaicism. *Prenatal Diagn* 1991;11:743–50

88. Verp MS, Unger NL. Placental chromosome abnormalities and intrauterine growth retardation (IUGR). *Proceedings of the 35th Annual Meeting of the Society for Gynecologic Investigation.* Baltimore, March, 1988:143

89. Stioui S, De Silvestris M, Molinari A, Stripparo L, Ghisoni L, Simoni G. Trisomic 22 placenta in a case of severe intrauterine growth retardation. *Prenat Diagn* 1989;9:673–6

90. Holzgreve B, Exeler R, Holzgreve W, Wittwer B, Miny P. Non-viable trisomies confined to the placenta leading to poor pregnancy outcome. *Prenat Diagn* 1992;12(Suppl May):95

91. Hashish AF, Monk NA, Lovell-Smith MP, Bardwell LM, Fiddes TM, Gardner RJM. Trisomy detected at chorionic villus sampling. *Prenat Diagn* 1989;9:427–32

92. Williams J, Wang B, Rubin C, Clark R, Oblandas T. Apparent non mosaic trisomy 16 in chorionic villi: diagnostic dilemma or clinically significant findings. *Am J Hum Genet* 1989;45A:273

93. Reddy NS, Blakemore KJ, Stetten G, Corson U. The significance of trisomy 7 mosaicism in chorionic villus cultures. *Prenat Diagn* 1990;10:417–23

94. Appelman Z, Rosensaft J, Cheuake J, et al. Trisomy 9 confined to the placenta: prenatal diagnosis and neonatal follow up. *Am J Med Genet* 1991;40:464–6

95. Tharapel T, Elias S, Shulman LP, Seely L, Emerson DS, Simpson JL. Resorbed co-twin as an explanation for discrepant chorionic villus results: non mosaic 47,XX, +16 in villi (direct and culture) with normal (46,XX) amniotic fluid and neonatal blood. *Prenat Diagn* 1989;9:467–72

96. Miny P, Hammer P, Gerlach B, et al. Mosaicism and accuracy of prenatal cytogenetic diagnoses after chorionic villus sampling and placental biopsies. *Prenat Diagn* 1991;11:581–9

97. Giles GW, Trudinger BJ, Baird PJ. Fetal umbilical artery flow velocity waveforms and placental resistance: a pathological correlation. *Br J Obstet Gynecol* 1985;92:31–8

98. Trudinger BJ, Cook CM. Umbilical and uterine artery flow velocity waveforms in pregnancy associated with major fetal abnormality. *Br J Obstet Gynaecol* 1985;92:666–70

99. Meizner I, Katz M, Lunenfeld E, Insler V. Umbilical and uterine flow velocity in pregnancies complicated by major fetal anomalies. *Prenat Diagn* 1987;7:491–3

100. Rankin JAG, McLaughlin MK. The regulation of placental blood flow. *J Dev Physiol* 1979;1:3–30

101. Campbell S, Pearce JMF, Hackett G, Cohen-Overbeek T, Hernández C. Quality assessment of uteroplacental blood flow early screening test for high-risk pregnancies. *Obstet Gynecol* 1986;68:649–53

102. Khons YT, Pearce JMF. Development and investigation of the placenta and its blood supply. In Lavery JP, ed. *The Human Placenta.* Rockeville, Maryland: Aspen, 1987:25–46

103. Shapiro BL. Down syndrome: a disruption of homeostasis. *Am J Med Genet* 1983;14:241–69

104. Jones CT. Reprogramming of metabolic development by restriction of fetal growth. *Biochem Soc Trans* 1985;13:84–91

105. Kornguth SE, Bersn ET, Auerbach R, Sobkowiez HM, Schutta HS, Scott GL. Trisomy 16 mice: neural, morphological and immunological studies. *Ann NY Acad Sci* 1986;477:160–78

106. Rochelson B, Kaplan C, Guzmán E, Arato M, Hausen K, Trunca C. A quantitative analysis of placental vasculature in the third trimester fetus with autosomal trisomy. *Obstet Gynecol* 1990;75:59–63

107. Hsieh FJ, Chang FM, Ko TM, Chen HY, Chen YP. Umbilical artery flow velocity waveforms in fetuses dying with congenital anomalies. *Br J Obstet Gynaecol* 1988;95:478–82

108. Hata K, Hazat D, Sendh D, Aoki S, Takamiya O, Kitao M. Umbilical artery blood flow velocity waveforms and association with fetal abnormality. *Ginecol Obstet Invest* 1989;27:179–82

109. Gaziano E, Knok E, Wager GP, et al. Pulsed Doppler umbilical artery waveforms: significance of elevated artery systolic/diastolic ratios in the normally grown fetus. *Obstet Gynecol* 1990;75:189–93

110. Carrera JM, Mortera C. Estudio Doppler de lso defectos congénitos. Abstracts I. *Congress of International Society of Ultrasound in Obstetrics and Gynaecology.* London: December 1991

111. Winick M, Noble A. Cellular response in rats during malnutrition at various ages. *J Nutr* 1966;89:300–6

112. Winick M, Coscia A, Noble A. Cellular growth of human placenta. I. Normal placental growth. *Pediatrics* 1967;39:248–51

113. Winick M. Changes in nucleic acid and protein content of the human brain during growth of the human brain. *Pediatr Res* 1968;2:352–5

114. Winick M, Rosso P. Head circumference and cellular growth of the brain in normal and marasmic children. *J Pediatr* 1969;74:774–8

115. Winick M, Brasel J, Rosso P. Nutrition and cell

growth. In Winick M, ed. *Nutrition and Development*. New York: John Wiley, 1972

116. Tajani N, Mann LI, Weiss RR. Antenatal diagnosis and management of the small-for-gestational-age fetus. *Obstet Gynecol* 1976;47:31

117. Hobbins JC. *Diagnostic Ultrasound in Obstetrics*. New York: Churchill Livingstone, 1979

118. Campbell S, Dewhurst CJ. Diagnosis of the small-for-dates fetus by serial ultrasonic cephalometry. *Lancet* 1971;2:1002–15

119. Campbell S, Thoms A. Ultrasound measurement of the fetal head to abdomen circumference ratio in the assessment of growth retardation. *Br J Obstet Gynaecol* 1977;84:165–79

120. Levi S, Kenwez J. Poor intrauterine fetal growth classification based on intrauterine echography. In Salvadori B, Bacchi-Modena A, eds. *Poor Intrauterine Fetal Growth*. Parma: Minerva Medica, 1977:37–41

121. Levi S, Maamari R. Ecographic diagnosis of PIFG. In Salvadori B, Bacchi-Modena A, eds. *Poor Intrauterine Fetal Growth*. Parma: Minerva Medica, 1977:251–4

122. Warsof SL, Cooper DJ, Little D, Campbell S. Routine ultrasound screening for antenatal detection of intrauterine growth retardation. *Obstet Gynecol* 1986;67:33–9

123. Clark SL. Patterns of intrauterine growth retardation. *Clin Obstet Gynecol* 1992;35:194–201

124. Rosso P, Winick M. Intrauterine growth retardation. A new systematic approach based on the clinical and biometrical characteristics of this condition. *J Perinatol Med* 1974;42:147–60

125. Sieroszewski J. Poor intrauterine fetal growth. Classification system for the fetus. In Salvadori B, Bacchi-Modena A, eds. *Poor Intrauterine Fetal Growth*. Parma: Minerva Medica, 1977:31–5

126. Holtorff J. Poor intrauterine fetal growth. An intrauterine nomenclature approach. In Salvadori B, Bacchi-Modena A, eds. *Poor Intrauterine Fetal Growth*. Parma: Minerva Medica, 1977:23–7

127. Miller RC, Hassanein K. Diagnosis of impaired fetal growth in newborn infants. *Pediatrics* 1971; 48:511–22

128. Villar J, Belizan JM. The timing factor in the pathophysiology of the intrauterine growth retardation syndrome. *Obstet Gynecol Surv* 1982; 37:499–506

129. Balcazar H, Haas J. Classification schemes of small-for-gestational age and type of intrauterine growth retardation and its implications to early neonatal mortality. *Early Hum Dev* 1990;24:219–30

130. Grauw TJ, Hopkins B. Severity of growth retardation and physical condition at birth in small for gestational age infants. *Biol Neonate* 1991;60:176–83

131. Tudehope DI. Neonatal aspects of intrauterine growth retardation. *Fetal Med Rev* 1991;3:73–85

132. Soothill PW, Bobrow CS, Holmes R. Small for gestational age is not a diagnosis. *Ultrasound Obstet Gynecol* 1999;13:225–8

133. Gruenwald P. Chronic fetal distress and placental insufficiency. *Biol Neonate* 1963;5:215–21

134. Carrera JM. Intrauterine growth retardation. *VIII World Congress of Gynecology and Obstetrics (FIGO)*, Mexico, October 1976

135. Carrera JM. Diagnóstico prenatal del retardo de crecimiento fetal. In *Clínica Ginecológica*, Vol. 2(3). Barcelona: Salvat, 1977

136. Carrera JM. Diagnosis of the intrauterine growth retardation. In Salvadori B, Bacchi-Modena A, eds. *Poor Intrauterine Fetal Growth*. Parma: Minerva Medica, 1977:277–81

137. Carrera JM. Concepto, selección y clasificación de los recién nacidos pequeños por retardo de crecimiento intrauterino. *Prog Obstet Ginecol* 1978; 21:197–208

138. Carrera JM, Mallafré J. Tratamiento <<in utero>> del retardo de crecimiento fetal. In Esteban Altirriba J, ed. *Perinatología Clínica*, Vol. 3. Barcelona: Salvat, 1980

139. Carrera JM. Regulación del crecimiento fetal. In Carrera JM, ed. *Biología y Ecología Fetal*. Barcelona: Salvat, 1981

140. Carrera JM. Crecimiento fetal: Sus alteraciones. In *Clínica Ginecológica*, Vol. 5(3). Barcelona: Salvat, 1981:1–7

141. Carrera JM. Patogénesis del crecimiento intrauterino retardado. In *Clínica Ginecológica*, Vol. 5(3). Barcelona: Salvat, 1981:71–85

142. Carrera JM, Serrat X. Crecimiento intrauterino retardado: Concepto, frecuencia y clasificación. In *Clínica Ginecológica*, Vol. 5(3). Barcelona: Salvat, 1981:36–42

143. Carrera JM. Clasificación del crecimiento intrauterino retardado. Doctoral thesis. Santiago de Compostela, 1981

144. Carrera JM. Tratamiento prenatal del retraso de crecimiento fetal. In Carrera JM, ed. *Biología y Ecología Fetal*. Barcelona: Salvat, 1981

145. Carrera JM, Serra B. Clasificación del crecimiento intrauterino retardado. *Rev Iberoam Fertil* 1993;10:21–30

146. Drugan A, Johnson MP, Isada NB, *et al*. The smaller than expected first trimester fetus if at increased risk for chromosome anomalies. *Am J Obstet Gynecol* 1992;167:1525–8

147. Weiner CP, Williamson RA. Evaluation of severe growth retardation using cordocentesis – hematologic and metabolic alterations by etiology. *Obstet Gynecol* 1989;73:225–9

148. Lockwood CJ, Weiner S. Assessment of fetal growth. *Clin Perinatol* 1986;13:3–35

Diagnosis of intrauterine growth restriction

4

J. M. Carrera, K. Maeda, C. Comas and M. Torrents

INTRODUCTION

In current clinical practice, with the introduction of ancillary explorations, namely ultrasound and other tests such as the non-stress test (NST), the biophysical profile and Doppler, it is possible to make many prenatal diagnoses:

(1) Risk for intrauterine growth restriction (IUGR);

(2) Screening for IUGR;

(3) Ultrasound diagnosis of IUGR;

(4) Type of IUGR;

(5) Fetal hemodynamics;

(6) Fetal assessment.

DIAGNOSIS OF THE RISK OF IUGR

Pregnancies at risk for IUGR may be diagnosed on the basis of previous history (e.g. low fetal birth weight in earlier pregnancies), associated disorders (e.g. autoimmune diseases, high blood pressure) and toxic habits (e.g. regular smoking). Previous history of IUGR is the most important risk factor[1,2]. Pregnancies with a two-fold or three-fold increased risk should be given special attention and fetal growth should be closely monitored[2-4].

Attempts have been made to predict the risk of IUGR, in particular in association with pregnancy-induced hypertension, using Doppler velocimetry in maternal uterine arteries. Campbell and associates[5] assessed arcuate artery velocity waveforms in low-risk pregnancies between weeks 16 and 18 of gestation, and reported a positive predictive value of 42%, negative predictive value of 87%, sensitivity of 68% and specificity of 69%. Steele and colleagues[6] obtained similar results. Nevertheless, other groups[7] have reported less encouraging data. In our opinion, the presence of a protodiastolic notch in uterine artery velocity waveforms that persists up to 25–26 weeks should alert the investigator to the possibility of IUGR, generally associated with pre-eclampsia (sensitivity 80%).

SCREENING FOR IUGR

This is perhaps the most important and the most difficult diagnosis to make when we consider that more than 50% of pregnancies are free of any associated conditions that would alert obstetricians to the possibility of IUGR.

Non-ultrasonic parameters

Apart from the patient's previous history, underlying diseases, poor weight gain or toxic habits, the discrepancy between gestational age and the size of the uterus is the most clearly indicative sign of IUGR.

Serial symphysis–fundal height measurement is the most acceptable method used for initial screening for IUGR. Westin[8,9] has developed diagrams of the increase in the height of the uterus from week 18 to week 43 of gestation. It was shown that about week 28 of gestation the IUGR group differed (1.2 ± 0.4 cm) significantly ($p < 0.01$) from that of neonates with adequate weight at birth, and these differences increased from week 36 on.

Effer[10] drew a centile curve divided into six areas. If a value fell within area 5 (between the 25th and the 10th centiles), this could be indicative of incipient IUGR and the patient should be submitted to close surveillance. If values fell within area 6 (below the 10th centile) IUGR was likely.

Since 1976, we also have used a similar curve drawn from our own data (predictive value: positive 60%, negative 96%). The results of this measurement are particularly useful until week 37 of gestation. Clearly, the method is not applicable to cases of twin pregnancies, hydramnios, etc.

Campbell and Soothill[11] compared the sensitivity of symphysis–fundal height with fetal abdominal circumference measurements (76% vs. 83%) and found that there was no statistically significant difference. These authors concluded that basic screening for IUGR should use symphysis–fundal height measurement, a procedure that had the advantage of being able to be carried out at each control, reserving ultrasound biometric data for those cases in which symphysis–fundal height fell below the 5th centile.

Nevertheless, the majority of authors are in agreement that patients whose symphysis–fundal height does fall below the 5th centile should subsequently undergo testing that will be able to identify fetuses that are at high risk for developing chronic fetal distress, such as Doppler study of the umbilical cord[12,13].

Ultrasound screening

Serial measurements of biparietal diameter

Initially, and still in many places, the biparietal diameter (BPD) was the only measurement that was routinely taken for the assessment of fetal growth. When pregnancy is normal, this parameter falls within the normal range and can be considered a representative indicator of the growth of other fetal organs and tissues, but when pregnancy is abnormal it may still fall within the normal range (head size is rarely affected in many cases of IUGR) although in this case it is not representative of the growth of other fetal structures. On the other hand, misdiagnoses have been made on many occasions in fetuses with marked brachycephaly or dolichocephaly or with syndromes causing microcephaly in association with normal development of the rest of the body. In addition, measurement of the BPD does not permit determination of fetal weight and height growth with acceptable reliability. The substitution of BPD by head circumference or cephalic area does not substantially improve the sensitivity of the method.

Measurement of biparietal diameter and length of the femur

With the purpose of improving the screening method, measurement of the length of the femur has been introduced. It has the advantage that it measures a component of fetal longitudinal growth and does not suffer the sudden flattening out characteristic of cephalic parameters at term, although it has the disadvantage of not being a useful parameter for establishing the diagnosis of IUGR at early stages.

Measurement of biparietal diameter, length of the femur and an abdominal parameter

The combination of these three parameters, if they are correctly measured, provides a considerably higher sensitivity than measurement of BPD alone or in association with the length of the femur. Inclusion of an abdominal parameter (abdominal diameter, abdominal circumference or abdominal area) adds a measurement that is earlier affected by growth restriction than cephalic or longitudinal development. An important limitation, however, is the high variability and low reproducibility of these measurements. Values within the normal or abnormal ranges may be found according to the section site.

Ultrasound screening of abnormal fetal growth is based on results of the three basic sonographic studies generally recognized as necessary in the control of a supposedly normal pregnancy, that is, at 8–12, 18–22 and 34–36 weeks of gestation. Measurement of the crown–rump length (CRL) is obtained in the first examination, so that gestational age is determined with notable accuracy, whereas other biometric parameters are measured on the second and third occasions of echographic study. Comparison of data obtained in both these examinations will permit identification of deviations from normality.

ULTRASOUND DIAGNOSIS OF IUGR

The diagnosis of IUGR is based on biometric parameters recorded during ultrasound scanning. For data to be useful, however, measurements must be standardized (precisely defined cross-sections for ultrasound imaging, clear reference points, etc.), discrimination consistent (identical cut-off points to differentiate fetuses and neonates) and appropriate curves used for the different populations under study which should then be correctly interpreted. It should be borne in mind that the independent variable, used to calculate the dependent variable, is located in the abscissa. In order to reduce misreadings to a minimum, gestational age should be precisely determined. If it is not clinically reliable, it must be determined by using measurements of fetal structures that are affected either little or not at all by fetal growth retardation, such as transverse cerebellar diameter[14–18].

Ultrasound parameters

Although there are multiple standardized measurements of fetal parameters for which tables or curves showing normal values have been developed, the following parameters are those used in clinical practice.

Crown–rump length

This is a particularly sensitive biometric parameter that can be measured in the early stages of gestation[19]. The greatest value of this parameter is the early confirmation of the gestational age, which, if measured in all gestations, allows for the early diagnosis of

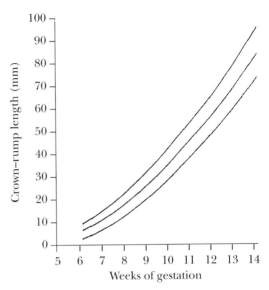

Figure 1 Mean ± 2 SD fetal crown–rump length for gestational age 6–14 weeks

IUGR. Technically the only limitation is the progressive bending of the embryo which makes measurements less reliable after weeks 10–12 of gestation. Between weeks 6–12 of gestation there is an exponential increase in CRL although this increase later appears to be linear. The maximum error obtained when calculating this parameter with respect to gestational age is ± 5 days in 95% of cases (between weeks 6 and 14, fetal growth is rapid and the limits of confidence are very narrow). If an embryo falls well outside the normal curve, the presence of chromosome anomalies or dysmorphy should be suspected. Fetal surveillance using ultrasound imaging should be instituted and the karyotype determined (Figure 1).

Biparietal diameter

This is the most reproducible parameter; it may be determined from weeks 13–14 of gestation (Figure 2). Many would consider this biometric parameter to be the most useful, not only to determine gestational age, but also to diagnose IUGR. Currently, this parameter is not used alone, but in conjunction with other biometric parameters.

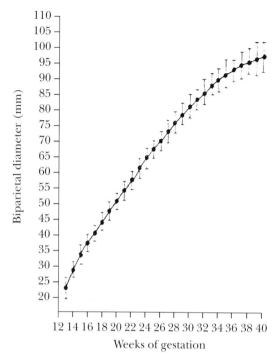

Figure 2 Relationship between biparietal diameter (mean ± 1 SD) and gestational age

The principal advantage of this measurement is the fact that it is relatively little affected by processes of nutritional deprivation or placental insufficiency, which permits it to be used, in spite of these conditions, for the determination of the probable gestational age.

The sonographic section, from front to back, includes[20] the most anterior portion of the longitudinal fissure, the cavum of the septum pellucidum, the thick line of the third ventricle and quadrigeminal cisterna with the punctiform echo on the pineal body. Frontal horns of the lateral ventricles and thalami on either side of the third ventricle should be visible[20,21].

Until week 30 of gestation, increases in BPD are reasonably linear, with weekly increases of 3 mm, approximately equal to the standard deviation of mean values for this period[22,23]. From weeks 30 to 38, the rate of change gradually slows, with weekly increases of about 1.5 mm[23,24]. From week 38 to term, weekly increases are 1 mm, and virtually nil as from week 42. The sum of the different rates of

increase in BPD causes standard deviations to increase as pregnancy reaches term.

Campbell and Dewhurst[25] reported that when the BPD was lower than the 5th centile, IUGR was confirmed in 68% of cases. Most errors occurred when values fell between the 5th and the 10th centiles; in these circumstances, weight at birth was within the normal range in 69% of newborns.

The sensitivity of the BPD as the only cephalometric parameter does not exceed 50%[26] (varying from 26.9% to 48%)[27–30] when determining a small-for-dates fetus below the 10th centile. In our experience, the sensitivity of the BPD between weeks 34 and 36 of gestation is 45% (Table 1).

Given the variability of the BPD (at least three different weeks may theoretically be ascribed to each value), serial measurements are recommended. Sabbagha and associates[31] proposed determining the so-called 'growth-adjusted sonar age' in order to determine sonar age precisely and to improve the prediction of IUGR. The ideal evolution of the 226 cases in which serial measurements of BPD were made (the first within the 24th week and the last after the 30th) on an original centile curve is shown in Figure 3.

An analysis of these data shows interesting findings.

(1) It would be exceptional for BPD values to fall, between weeks 21 and 30, below the fiducial limits, provided that there were no date error, and the age were adjusted to BPD growth according to the method described by Sabbagha and colleagues[31];

(2) Only in 34.9% of all growth-adjusted sonar age by ultrasonography did the BPD fall below the 5th centile at some stage during pregnancy. Only by raising the band to the 25% mark did it prove possible to discriminate 83.62% of confirmed IUGR;

(3) In 16.7% of cases the BPD measurements were found above the 25% mark;

(4) Theoretically, it is possible to determine fetal growth models. Each model has a

Table 1 Comparison of several biometric parameters for detection of the small-for-gestational-age infant at 34 or 36 weeks of gestation

	Sensitivity	Specificity	Predictive value	
			Positive	Negative
Biparietal diameter	45	74.5	23.0	81.5
Cephalic circumference	52	80.0	26.0	94.3
Cephalic area	60	80.0	23.0	95.2
Abdominal circumference	83	87.7	43.0	97.8
Abdominal area	85	88.0	44.0	98.1
Femur length	58	81.0	23.3	95.0

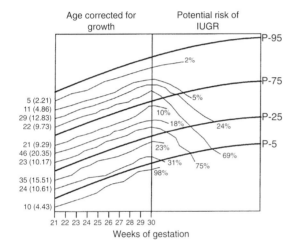

Figure 3 Potential risk of intrauterine growth restriction (IUGR) according to the evolution of biparietal diameter (BPD). Curves are shown for the 5th, 25th, 75th and 95th centiles, with 'small', 'medium' and 'large' BPD between them. Numbers of cases analyzed[31] are shown on the left, with percentage incidence of IUGR in parentheses. The potential risk of IUGR is shown on the right

determined relative incidence (on the left of the figure) and a different potential risk of IUGR (on the right of the figure).

At present, despite the fact that it continues to be the most frequently used biometric parameter, the BPD is not considered to be a reliable indicator of IUGR. This is because head size is rarely affected in many cases of IUGR (in particular type II IUGR, the most commonly occurring) and, moreover,

because in the last weeks of pregnancy it is very difficult to determine whether or not the fetus is really growing, since weekly gains in fetal weight are minimal. On the other hand, the BPD should be used when the cephalic index (fronto-occipital diameter divided by BPD and multiplied by 100) falls between 70 and 85.

Differential diagnosis between IUGR and 'miscalculation of estimated day of delivery'

When the BPD is apparently below the lower limits of confidence, it does not necessarily signify IUGR. There may be an error in the calculation of the estimated day of delivery.

The possibility of an error in the estimated day of delivery can be eliminated by performing an ultrasound examination in the first trimester of gestation (data from the size of the embryo or yolk sac). The diagnosis of IUGR is especially consistent when cephalic measurements are initiated early. If the cephalic curve remains parallel to the standard curve throughout the gestation, then we are dealing with a pregnancy with earlier dates. In contrast, if we are dealing with IUGR, the curve will deviate from the theoretical standard curve at a given moment during the gestation.

Nevertheless, it is not always possible to have early measurements to observe the exact moment at which a fetus begins to deviate from the standard growth curve. In practice, we need to resort to the method of weekly increments. We are indebted to Campbell and Newman[32], who performed serial studies of fetal growth and have established graphs in which the relationship of weekly growth, BPD and gestational age are demonstrated.

It is thus possible to determine in successive weekly measurements whether, in a given case, the weekly growth of the fetus is adequate. In contrast, one can ascertain the gestational age using the data from the weekly increase in growth. If one is dealing with a questionable date of the last menstrual period (LMP), a suspicion for IUGR will arise in any fetus whose weekly increase in the measurement of the BPD is below the 10th centile of the expected measurement and it can almost be confirmed for any increase that is lower than the 5th centile.

If there are any doubts of the LMP or if the expected BPD is less than that expected for a given gestational age, one can resort to the second graph, which permits the evaluation of the increments as a function of the BPD. If the weekly increments remain below those expected for a given BPD, it is most probable that one is dealing with a fetus with IUGR, especially if the weekly increase is below the 5th centile. If the measurements agree, then one is dealing with a miscalculation of the gestational age.

Head circumference and/or cephalic area

Measuring the head circumference or cephalic area is a more complex procedure than measuring BPD since, for measurements to be correct, the sonographic section should include both the biparietal and the fronto-occipital diameters. These parameters, however, have some advantages over the BPD, since they avoid the errors that occur in BPD measurements as a result of brachycephaly or dolichocephaly (e.g. craniosynostosis); and in cases of breech presentation, which often accompanies a fundic placenta, BPD measurements in normally developed fetuses are abnormally small, while head circumference or cephalic area are within normal limits (Figure 4).

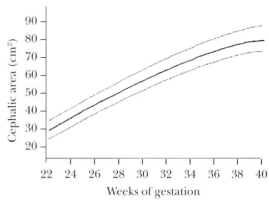

Figure 4 Relationship between cephalic area (mean ± 2 SD) and gestational age

The sensitivity of head circumference measurements is 52% and, therefore, somewhat higher than that of BPD. Specificity, however, is similar (80%). Predictive values do not seem to differ greatly whether head circumference or cephalic area are used. In our experience (using our own curve) the sensitivity of cephalic area is 60% and specificity 80% (Table 1).

Abdominal diameters

Both transverse and anteroposterior abdominal diameters have been used to assess fetal development. Some authors[33,34] consider that measurement of abdominal diameters has the advantage over abdominal circumference or abdominal area of being much simpler and open to fewer errors. To ensure the reproducibility of abdominal diameter measurements:

(1) A cross-sectional view should be obtained from the appropriate site (the site of choice is the level at which the umbilical vein leads into the canal of Arantius (ductus venosus). At this point the diameter of the fetal liver and, therefore, of the abdomen is at its greatest;

(2) The section should be as close to orthogonal as possible;

(3) The measurement should be made during a moment of fetal apnea.

Macler and co-workers[33], correlating false-positive and false-negative results from the BPD, thoracic diameter and abdominal diameter, have shown that figures were particularly low, throughout gestation, when abdominal diameters were used.

Abdominal circumference or abdominal area

These parameters are considered to be the best indicators of fetal growth, since they reflect the volume of an important complete organ, such as the fetal liver. On the other hand, by comparing them to cephalic parameters, it allows for the phenotypic type of IUGR to be determined.

Measurement of the abdominal circumference or abdominal area of the fetus is facilitated by the cylindrical shape of this body segment and the existence of an excellent point of reference (the umbilical vein). The curve of values for the abdominal circumference during pregnancy shows an almost linear increase until week 36, with a slight decrease from this time on. The tendency for values to fall off suddenly at term, typical of cephalometric parameters, is, therefore, not detected (Figure 5).

If measurements of abdominal circumference are compared with those of head circumference it may be observed that, although mean abdominal circumference measurements are at first smaller than mean head circumference measurements, they equal out at week 36, and from then on the mean abdominal circumference measurements are greater than those of head circumference. According to Campbell and Wilkin[35] the diagnostic accuracy of this parameter in cases of IUGR is remarkable; using a single measurement at week 32 of gestation, 86.7% of newborns who fall below the 5th centile can be identified. Results are less favorable, however, as pregnancy progresses. At weeks 35 to 36, Campbell and Soothill[11] reported a sensitivity of 83%, specificity of 79%, positive predictive value of 39% and negative predictive value of 87%. Similar results have been reported by other authors[36,37]. In our experience this parameter showed an overall sensitivity of 83% with a

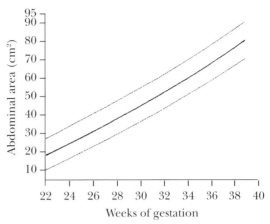

Figure 5 Relationship between abdominal area (mean ± 2 SD) and gestational age

specificity of 87.7%; in the case of abdominal area, the sensitivity and specificity were 85% and 88%, respectively[38].

It should be noted that sensitivity and positive predictive value increase with gestational age, so that week 34 ± 1 of pregnancy is considered to be the best time for differentiating fetuses with IUGR[39,40].

Unfortunately, both head circumference and head area measurements are subject to greater inter- and intraobserver variations than BPD, owing to the changes that take place in measurements as a result of fetal breathing movements and fetal position[41].

Length of femur

The femur is the easiest long bone to identify and measure. On the other hand, it offers an advantage over the BPD since it does not change with morphological changes of the fetal head, and it also permits the evaluation of certain types of skeletal dysplasias. Its typical 'golf club'-like appearance and moderate curvature from week 18 on are unmistakable. The normal curve for length of femur, similar to that of abdominal parameters, does not suffer the sudden flattening out characteristic of cephalic parameters (Figure 6).

O'Brien and Queenan[42,43] showed that fetal femur length values in 60% of cases of IUGR fell below the lower confidence limit. This parameter, just like cephalic parameters, is

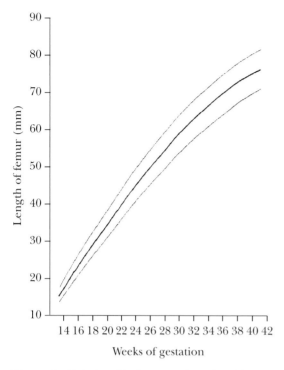

Figure 6 Relationship between length of femur (mean ± 2 SD) and gestational age

affected in cases of symmetrical fetal growth retardation (type I) but is hardly or not at all affected in cases of asymmetrical fetal growth retardation (type II). Hadlock and colleagues[44] have emphasized the usefulness of the femur length/abdominal circumference ratio, which not only presents acceptable levels of sensitivity (63%) but also has the advantage of being independent of gestational age. Indeed, this ratio remains constant (22 ± 2%) as from week 22 of gestation. Its predictive value, however, is less than 30%[45].

Diagnosis from the delay of the growth of BPD and femur length

The pregnancy weeks matched to the sizes of sonographic fetal parameters are calculated, and compared to actual pregnancy weeks calculated from the CRL in the first trimester or reliable LMP. A common manual method is to compare the measured BPD and femur length to the growth curves of the BPD and femur length standardized in each district or region. It will be appropriate, for example, in Japan to use femur length growth values reported by the Japanese Society of Obstetrics and Gynecology[46], where fetal femur length value is smaller than the European standard in late pregnancy.

A computerized technique is to calculate the pregnancy weeks from the values of BPD and/or femur length (Table 2). IUGR is suggested, if the pregnancy weeks determined by the computer programs repeatedly delay in the third trimester from the weeks determined by the CRL or correct LMP.

Total intrauterine volume

Gohari and co-workers[47] have measured maximum longitudinal (L), transverse (T) and anteroposterior (AP) diameters of the uterus to calculate total intrauterine volume (TIUV) (TIUV = L × T × AP × 0.5233). Using measurements obtained from 100 pregnancies at different stages of gestation, they calculated a normal curve. In a series of 96 cases of suspected IUGR (with postnatal confirmation in 28 cases), it was concluded that IUGR is likely when total intrauterine volume corresponds to –1.5 SD of the mean, equivocal when figures fall between –1.5 and +1.5 SD of the mean (one-third of cases of IUGR), or should be excluded when they are over –1 SD. The only errors recorded were those caused by severe oligohydramnios. Results of some later studies, however, are less encouraging (sensitivity 60%, positive predictive value 30%)[30].

Fetal organs biometry

Currently we study the biometry of certain organs (diameters, estimation of volume, etc.) of diverse fetal organs such as the brain, the heart, the lungs, the liver, the spleen, the pancreas, the stomach, the suprarenal glands, the intestine and the bladder[48]. Nevertheless, in general, and with the exception of measuring the volume of the bladder to calculate the production of urine by the fetus, these parameters have little value in diagnosing IUGR.

Table 2 BASIC computer program for the estimation of the weeks of pregnancy from fetal biparietal diameter (BPD) or femur length (FL). "PREGNANCY" shows the center value of the weeks (W) and days (D) of pregnancy, and "RANGES: DW ED-HW LD" indicates the ranges of possible weeks and days of pregnancy. × is the multiplication sign

```
690:   PRINT "BPD OR FL & GEST WEEKS/ MAEDA & IWAMOTO": REM 1984
692:   INPUT "BY BPD=1, FEMUR=0, ENTER" Y: IF Y<1 THEN 715
693:   INPUT "BPD(MM)=; X: IF X<20 THEN 745
694:   IF X>94 THEN 745
695:   IF X<79 THEN 705
700:   W=1063.378-23.671 × X+X² × 0.1615: Y=1132.136-25.28 × X+X² × 0.173
702:   Z=1260.348-28.227 × X+X² × 0.192: GOSUB 740: GOTO 707
705:   W=37.181+1.849 × X+X² × 0.0027: Y= 42.315+1.807 × X+X² × 0.0045
706:   Z=47.448+1.78 × X+X² × 0.006: GOSUB 740
707:   PRINT "PREGNANCY ";F; "W"; G; "D"
710:   PRINT RANGES: "; D; "W"; E; "D-"; H; "W"; I; "D"; END
715:   INPUT "FEMUR LENGTH (MM)=";X: IF X>72 THEN 745
720:   IF X<15 THEN 745
725:   IF X<61 THEN 735
730:   W=415.445-9.417 × X+X² × 0.103: Y=508.462-12.108 × X+X² × 0.125
732:   Z=601.473-14.799 × X+X² × 0.147: GOSUB 740:GOTO 707
735:   W=58.4+2.286 × X+X² × 0.006: Y=63.164+2.272 × X²+0.008
737:   Z=67.927+22.258 × X+X² × 0.01: GOSUB 740: GOTO 707
740:   D=INT(W/7): E=INT(W-D × 7): F=INT(Y/7): G=INT(Y-F × 7): H=INT(Z/7):
       I=INT(Z-H × 7): RETURN
745:   PRINT "VALUE IS OUT OF RANGE"
750    END
```

Examples of calculation. Italic number shows the key input:

(1) BPD OR FL & GEST WEEKS/ MAEDA & IWAMOTO
    BY BPD=1, FEMUR=0, ENTER *1*
    BPD (MM) = *63*
    PREGNANCY 24W 6D
    RANGES: 23W 3D-26W 1D

(2) BPD OR FL & GEST WEEKS/ MAEDA & IWAMOTO
    BY BPD=1, FEMUR=0, ENTER *1*
    BPD (MM) = *94*
    PREGNANCY 40W 4D
    RANGES: 37W 6D-43W 2D

(3) BPD OR FL & GEST WEEKS/ MAEDA & IWAMOTO
    BY BPD=1, FEMUR=0, ENTER *0*
    FEMUR LENGTH (MM) = *46*
    PREGNANCY 26W 2D
    RANGES: 25W 1D-27W 3D

(4) BPD OR FL & GEST WEEKS/ MAEDA & IWAMOTO
    BY BPD=1, FEMUR=0, ENTER *0*
    FEMUR LENGTH (MM)= *65*
    PREGNANCY 35W 4D
    RANGES: 34W 0D-37W 1D

Estimated fetal body weight

Fetal body weight is estimated from sonographic parameters, and compared to a standard fetal body weight curve standardized in the district or region. IUGR is diagnosed when the estimated fetal weight (EFW) is lower than the 5th centile of the standard value in the pregnancy weeks determined by CRL in the first trimester or correct LMP. Continuously lower EFW than the 10th centile of the standard curve also suggests the presence of IUGR. Restricted growth or fetal malnutrition mainly due to placental abnormality will be assessed by other analyses, particularly the ratio of head circumference to abdominal circumference (HC/AC ratio). Fetal growth restriction will be diagnosed when the HC/AC ratio is high, and higher than unity in the stage after 35 weeks of pregnancy.

Formulae of fetal weight estimation and the computer program

Various formulae have been reported for the processing of sonographic parameters, including diameters, circumferences and areas, in the estimation of fetal body weight. Campbell and Silkin (1975)[49] used the following formula:

$$\log_e (EFW) = -4.564 + 0.282(AC) - 0.00331(AC^2)$$

Hadlock and colleagues (1985)[50] used the following, in which FDL stands for femoral diaphysis length:

(1) $\log_{10} (EFW) = 1.304 + 0.05281(AC) + 0.1938(FDL) - 0.004(AC \times FDL)$

(2) $\log_{10} (EFW) = 1.335 + 0.0316(BPD) + 0.0457(AC) + 0.1623(FDL) - 0.0034(AC \times FDL)$

(3) $\log_{10} (EFW) = 1.326 + 0.0107(HC) + 0.0438(AC) + 0.158(FDL) - 0.00326(AC \times FDL)$

(4) $\log_{10} (FDL) = 1.3596 + 0.0064(HC) + 0.0424(AC) + 0.174(FDL) + 0.00061(BPD \times AC) - 0.00386(AC \times FDL)$

Shepard and co-workers(1982)[51] used the following:

$$\log_{10} (EFW) = -1.7492 + 0.166(BPD) + 0.046(AC) - 0.002546 (BPD \times AC)$$

Rose and McCallum (1987)[52] used the following, in which AD stands for abdominal diameter:

$$\log_e (EFW) = 4.2581 + 0.193 (BPD + AD)$$

$$\log_e (EFW) = 4.198 + 0.143 (BPD + AD + FDL)$$

Some investigators divided the fetal body into two spheres, calculated the volume of each, and multiplied the sum of the two by the average specific gravity of the fetus. The EFW was obtained as follows by Aoki and Ogata (1982)[53]:

$$EFW = 1.25647(BPD^3) + 3.50667(AC \times FL) + 6.30994 \tag{1}$$

The EFW was obtained as follows by Shinozuka (1987)[54]:

$$EFW = 1.07(BPD^3) + 3.42(APD \times TD \times FL) \tag{2}$$

FL, femur length; APD, abdominal antero-posterior diameter; TD, transverse diameter.

These formulae are commonly used in Japan, and their usefulness has been confirmed.

These equations will be used in computer programs for automated EFW determination. For example, equation (2) was programmed in BASIC by the author, and appropriate EFW values are demonstrated under the title 'FETAL WEIGHT' on the computer display at 18–40 weeks of pregnancy (Table 3).

EFW is automatically demonstrated on the sonographic screen in many commercial machines by the input of sonographic parameters and by the processing of equations of fetal body weight estimation.

Fetal volume is obtained by the summation of all transverse section areas multiplied by the average distance of each section obtained by ultrasonic scanning of the fetal body in the procedure of three-dimensional ultrasound. The volume is multiplied by the specific gravity of the fetus, allowing the most correct EFW to be obtained.

Table 3   The authors' BASIC computer program for the estimation of fetal weight by biparietal diameter (BPD), fetal abdominal anteroposterior diameter (APD), transverse diameter (TD) and femur length (FL). Original equation (fetal weight = $1.07 \times BPD^3 + 3.42 \times APD \times TD \times FL$, Shinozuka, 1987) is used in Japan. FL value is modified by the regression equation of FL and BPD, and input instead of BPD (Maeda, see text), when BPD measurement is difficult or fetal head is distorted. $\times$ is the multiplication sign

500:	INPUT "FETAL WEIGHT: USE BPD? YES=1 NO=0";X:IF X<1 THEN 520
510:	INPUT "BPD(MM)=";B: B=B/10
520:	INPUT "APD(MM)="; A: INPUT "TD(MM)="; T: INPUT "FL (MM)="; F: A=A/10: T=T/10: F=F/10: IF X<1 THEN 540
530:	INPUT "BPD(MM)="; B: B=B/10: Y=$1.07 \times B^3$+$3.42 \times A \times F \times T$: PRINT "FETAL WEIGHT="; INT(Y+0.5); "G" :END
540:	H=$1.156 \times F$+1.26: Y=$1.07 \times H^3$+$3.42 \times A \times F \times T$: PRINT "WEIGHT (NO BPD)="; INT(Y+0.5); "G" :END

Examples of computer calculation. "FETAL WEIGHT" was calculated by the use of BPD, and "WEIGHT (NO BPD)" was obtained by the exclusion of BPD (the percentage in the parenthesis indicates the error in the weight obtained by the use of BPD):

(1)   (18 weeks)
BPD (MM) = *42*
APD (MM) = *39*
TD (MM) = *43*
FL (MM) = *25*
FETAL WEIGHT= 223 G
WEIGHT (NO BPD)= 220 G (1.3%)

(2)   (22 weeks)
BPD (MM) = *56*
APD (MM) = *54*
TD (MM) = *56*
FL (MM) = *36*
FETAL WEIGHT= 560 G
WEIGHT (NO BPD)=543 G (3.0%)

(3)   (26 weeks)
BPD (MM) = *67*
APD (MM) = *64*
TD (MM) = *69*
FL (MM) = *49*
FETAL WEIGHT= 1062 G
WEIGHT (NO BPD)= 1095 G (3.1%)

(4)   (33 weeks)
BPD (MM) = *86*
APD (MM) = *96*
TD (MM) = *72*
FL (MM) = *60*
FETAL WEIGHT= 2099 G
WEIGHT (NO BPD)=2007 G (4.4%)

(5)   (34 weeks)
BPD (MM) = *85*
APD (MM) = *78*
TD (MM) = *100*
FL (MM) = *61*
FETAL WEIGHT= 2284 G
WEIGHT (NO BPD)= 2242 G (1.8%)

(6)   (35 weeks)
BPD (MM) = *83*
APD (MM) = *85*
TD (MM) = *99*
FL (MM) = *66*
FETAL WEIGHT= 2511 G
WEIGHT (NO BPD)=2651 G (5.6%)

(7)   (38 weeks)
BPD (MM) = *88*
APD (MM) = *99*
TD (MM) = *82*
FL (MM) = *63*
FETAL WEIGHT= 2478 G
WEIGHT (NO BPD)=2416 G (2.5%)

(8)   (40 weeks)
BPD (MM) = *93*
APD (MM) = *107*
TD (MM) = *108*
FL (MM) = *71*
FETAL WEIGHT= 3667 G
WEIGHT (NO BPD)=3714 G (1.3%)

Estimation of fetal weight by femur length and fetal abdominal diameters

The BPD is excluded in the calculation of EFW, when the BPD measurement is difficult because of deep descent into the pelvis, the shape of the fetal head is atypical with a long anteroposterior diameter, the fetal head is distorted, etc. Ferrero and colleagues[55] reported the equation without the use of BPD:

$$\log_{10}(EFW) = 0.77125 + 0.13244(AC)$$
$$- 0.12996(FL)$$
$$- 1.73588(AC^2)/1000$$
$$+ 3.09212(FL \times AC)/1000$$
$$+ 2.18984(FL/AC)$$

where r^2 was 0.987.

The authors found close correlation between BPD and femur length in their standard values reported by the Japanese Society of Obstetrics and Gynecology[46]. The regression equation of BPD and FL is: BPD = 1.158(FL) + 1.26 (cm), and the correlation coefficient (r^2) was 0.998 in nine periods ranging from 20 to 37 weeks of pregnancy. Therefore, the authors used the [1.158(FL) + 1.26] value instead of BPD in the programming of equation (2), and the results calculated by abdominal APD, TD and FL demonstrated only a small difference from the EFW estimated from BPD, APD, TD and FL (Table 3). Maeda wrote a BASIC computer program from equation (2) without the BPD, and applied it in clinical practice (Table 3). Study of this technique will be continued in a large field study after this preliminary report.

DIAGNOSIS OF TYPE OF IUGR

The prenatal knowledge of the biometric type of IUGR does not have the same importance as it did several years ago, when it was considered that symmetric IUGR was most probably associated with chromosomal or genetic abnormalities, and asymmetric IUGR with a vascular insufficiency of the uteroplacenatal bed. Recent studies have shown that chromosomal abnormalities can be associated with both types of IUGR[56,57] and that the asymmetry is a progressive phenomenon closely related to clinical severity in the restriction of fetal growth[58].

The prenatal diagnosis is fundamentally based on patient history and clinical information, the echographic findings and, to a lesser degree, on the prenatal testing that evaluates the fetal condition. The echographic identification of the type of IUGR is based on three evaluations:

(1) A profile of the cranial parameters;

(2) Calculation of the HC/AC ratio;

(3) Calculation of the diameter of the fetal thigh.

While the first measurement attempts to determine the precociousness of the growth retardation, the other two measurements are reflective of the nutritional status of the fetus.

Profile of the curve of cephalometric parameters

These data (BPD, head circumference or cephalic area) provide information on the moment when the noxa began to affect fetal cranial structures, thus distinguishing between fetal growth restriction of early (type I), late (type II) or semi-early (type III) onset.

In the case of type I IUGR (symmetrical or intrinsic), the curve of the mean values falls below −2 SD early in pregnancy and continues largely parallel to the latter. This is due to the fact that the noxa or the different noxae responsible for fetal growth retardation negatively influence, early and simultaneously, the three parameters that define growth – fetal length, fetal weight and head circumference.

In contrast, in type II IUGR (asymmetrical or extrinsic), the mean curve of BPD or head circumference coincides with mean values for the normal population until approximately week 30 of gestation, when it falls below the mean. Nevertheless, although it continues to decrease until the end of pregnancy, at no time does the mean of the affected group fall below −2 SD of mean values of the normal population. In this case, factors causing IUGR have exerted their influence late in the second trimester of pregnancy and, therefore, although they have had sufficient time to affect fetal nutrition, cranial structures that are much less susceptible to under-nourishment are affected little and late. In contrast, the rest of the fetal body soon suffers from undernourishment, with weight, height and thoracic and abdominal perimeters being primarily affected.

Finally, in type III IUGR (semi-harmonious), which usually results from maternal malnutrition, the BPD profile shows an intermediate pattern.

Calculation of the HC/AC ratio

The study of this ratio provides data on overall fetal morphology, helping to define fetal growth as proportionate (type I), disproportionate (type II) or semi-proportionate (type III). A relationship may be established between head and abdominal circumferences, diameters or areas.

The HC/AC ratio decreases throughout pregnancy[24] (values > 1.2 at 14 to 16 weeks; < 1 after 36 weeks; between 0.9 and 1 at term), owing to the rapid accumulation of fat in subcutaneous and soft tissues in the fetal thorax and abdomen during the last trimester.

Kurjak and Breyer[59] have the HC/AC ratio with the position of the newborn on the centile curve at 36 weeks. When this method was reproduced by our group, similar results were obtained, with the only difference being that, in the group of neonates below the 10th centile, one-third of cases showed a ratio of < 1, whereas in the experience of Kurjak and Breyer[59] this occurred in only 5% of infants in this group (Figure 7).

It may be concluded that the HC/AC ratio is inverted after week 36 of gestation (from > 1 to < 1). Only 7% of normal fetuses do not show this pattern[2].

Fetuses small for gestational age behave differently depending upon the causes of growth retardation. If the ratio is inverted and, therefore, values are within the confidence interval of the normal curve, it is safe to assume that the case is one of fetal growth retardation of the proportionate or

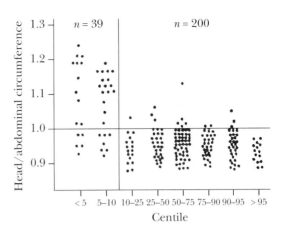

Figure 7 Relationship between the ratio of head/abdominal circumference and the position of the newborn on the centile curve at 36 weeks of gestation

symmetrical type (type I IUGR). The neonate that is small for gestational age is hypoplastic but not hypotrophic. Only 11.76% of infants do not show this pattern. Fetal growth retardation, however, will not go unnoticed at the time of sonographic examination since, as we have already mentioned, BPD is markedly affected. On the other hand, however, when the ratio is above the upper limit of the confidence interval of this curve and, consequently, is not inverted, the case is probably one of growth retardation of the asymmetrical, disproportionate or extrinsic type (IUGR type II) as a result of which newborn infants will be small for gestational age, hypotrophic and, in some cases, dystrophic. Only 7.14% of infants do not show this pattern[2]. Finally, in the case of IUGR type III (semi-proportionate), the ratio is > 1 in 41.7% cases, < 1 in 52.94% and equal to 1 in 5.82%.

In spite of the prenatal assignment of IUGR to one type or another, the prognostic importance of this has diminished in comparison to the situation several years ago. It is evident, nonetheless, that the diagnostic importance echographically of the HC/AC ratio means that it is a measurement that should be taken into account when determining the well-being of the fetus. As can be seen in Table 4, which demonstrates the experience of David and colleagues[58], there are differences that are

Table 4 Clinical data of the two subsets of small-for-gestational-age fetuses. The head-to-abdomen ratio was considered abnormal when it was > 2 standard deviations above the mean. Numerical variables are reported as mean ± 1 standard deviation. From reference 58

	Abnormal ratio (n = 56)	Normal ratio (n = 78)	Statistical analysis
Gestational age at delivery (weeks)	34 ± 3.6	36.3 ± 3.6	$p^* < 0.005$
Birth weight (g)	1533 ± 635	2022 ± 655	$p^\dagger < 0.0001$
Delta birth weight	−2.62 ± 10.73	−2.10 ± 0.67	$p^\dagger < 0.0001$
Abnormal UA Doppler	29 (52%)	20 (26%)	OR‡ 3.11 (1.14–6.92)
Abnormal biophysical profile	15 (27%)	9 (11%)	OR‡ 2.80 (1.04–7.73)
Emergency Cesarean section	21 (37%)	23 (29%)	OR‡ 1.43 (0.65–3.17)
Delivery at < 34 weeks**	19 (34%)	10 (13%)	OR‡ 3.49 (1.36–9.08)
Perinatal mortality	12 (21%)	6 (8%)	OR‡ 3.27 (1.04–9.34)
Chromosomal abnormalities	2	2	

UA, umbilical artery; *probability level derived from Mann–Whitney U test; †probability level derived from Student's t test; ‡odds ratio with 95% confidence interval; **excluding intrauterine deaths

statistically significant in the use of various parameters, depending on whether a given ratio is normal or elevated. In both groups, there could be deterioration of the fetal condition, but this possibility is obviously greater in the group of fetuses with IUGR with an elevated HC/AC ratio because, as previously stated, in this case the pathological restriction of ponderal growth is greater.

Fetal thigh diameter or perimeter

The quantity and distribution of fat present in the fetus is, without a doubt, one of the most significant parameters that represents the nutritional status of the fetus[60]. Even when this factor is evaluated indirectly by measuring the abdominal perimeter or area, and calculating the HC/AC ratio, it is evident that the proportion of fat in the fetal extremities, and especially in the thigh, is greater than in the abdomen[61–63]. It must be kept in mind, on the other hand, that the decrease in the abdominal parameters in the presence of asymmetric IUGR is not only due to the loss of fat, but also, and especially, due to the poor development of the liver.

Balouet and colleagues[64] have systematically calculated the cutaneous perimeter and aponeurosis of the thigh, proposing a formula to estimate fetal weight that, in addition, takes into account the umbilical perimeter. By this formula, the global precision was 6%, the correlation with fetal weight 0.954 and, in 82% of cases, the margin of error was less than 10%.

The confirmation of normal values should lead one to believe that the fetus is well nourished (if one is dealing with IUGR, it is most likely type I) and values that are obviously pathological should lead to a diagnosis of type II IUGR. Apparently, this procedure is efficacious in all fetal weights and varies little with ethnic conditions.

Complementary explorations in early IUGR

A notable contingent of the fetuses that are included in this group are those that have chromosomal abnormalities (Turner syndrome, various trisomies) or those with grave congenital abnormalities. All these infants have a reduction in the number of cells[65]. On the other hand, serious transplacental infections, such as rubella, cytomegalovirus or toxoplasmosis, can produce embryonic pathology. Finally, some of the fetuses in this group have poor stature by virtue of being dwarfs (Russell or Silver type dwarfism or achondroplastic dwarfism).

In those cases that are diagnosed as precocious or semi-precocious cases of IUGR, it is advisable to carry out further studies of the fetus to establish the existence of an anomaly or malformation of sufficient gravity to alter the obstetric care of the patient. It is especially important to evaluate whether a congenital defect or an embryonic infectious pathology exists.

Diagnosis of congenital defects

At present, the high definition of the latest echographic equipment allows for the prenatal diagnosis of the majority of malformations. The introduction of transvaginal ultrasound facilitates even earlier diagnosis (12–16 weeks) of a notable number of cases, especially those with poor prognosis. The use of three-dimensional techniques improves our diagnostic capabilities even more.

On the other hand, the three major trisomies (21, 18 and 13) are associated to a greater or lesser degree with IUGR, so that trisomy 18, for example, has been considered exemplary of symmetric IUGR. It has become recognized[66] that each of these trisomies presents its own model of somatic and visceral growth. As a gold standard or model, they can be suspected echographically if the expected growth curve for each aneuploidy is known and careful biometric studies are performed. In this regard, the studies by Barr[66] carried out in specimens of these trisomies during the second trimester of gestation have been very useful.

Suspicion for early IUGR, and a profile of pathological growth (a deprivation in all of the biometric parameters, but especially in the length of the extremities) should oblige one to perform a meticulous global morphological study looking for characteristic anomalies of each of these aneuploidies.

Finally, we currently rely upon the collection of fetal material at any point in gestation beyond 9–10 weeks: amniocentesis, chorionic villus sampling, funiculocentesis, etc. This allows us to determine the fetal karyotype and assess whether or not a chromosomal abnormality exists.

Immunological screening for infectious diseases

Maternal serological screening permits the selection of gravid women who are at risk of developing a certain infection, or women who have already developed a given infection. The goal of this screening is to demonstrate whether an infection is currently present, or has been present in the past. The diagnostic algorithm to detect whether the fetus has been infected includes the following steps.

Diagnosis of the maternal infection   There is no need to determine whether the fetus has been infected without prior confirmation of maternal infection. The diagnosis can be clinical (when the symptoms are evident) or serological. For the serological diagnosis, it is fundamental to determine the presence of IgG or IgM antibodies that are specific to the corresponding virus or parasite. The algorithm demonstrated in Figure 8 summarizes the serological process necessary to confirm maternal infection with the TORCH viruses. Once the maternal infection is confirmed, the next step is to rule out possible fetal infection.

Diagnosis of fetal infection   Maternal infection is not necessarily followed by fetal infection. As is well known, IgG easily crosses the placental barrier, whereas IgM does not, owing to its high molecular weight. It has been proven that the fetus begins to synthesize IgM after 15–16 weeks, although until 19–20 weeks the concentration of this class of antibody is not sufficient to be easily detected. Until recently, the only routine technique that was at our disposal to evaluate specific IgM antibodies in the fetus was through blood obtained by cordocentesis. The amount of specific IgM noted should be negative; if it is positive, one should suspect the presence of a fetal infection, which will be confirmed if the infectious agent is diagnosed by means of DNA hybridization techniques. Nowadays, detection by the

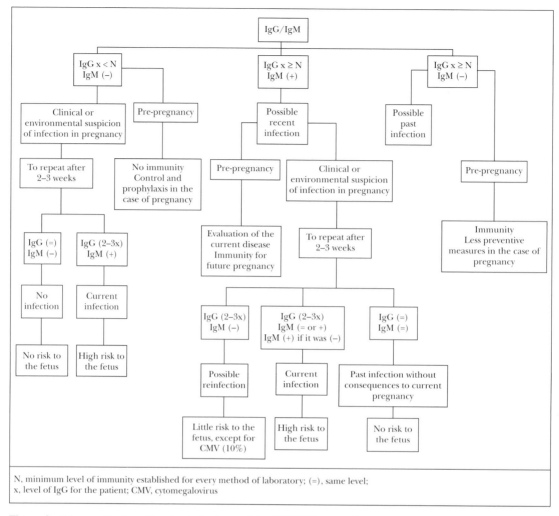

Figure 8 Diagnostic algorithm for infections of the TORCH group in pregnant women

polymerase chain reaction (PCR) in amniotic fluid is also used.

In certain infections, such as cytomegalovirus, before performing cordocentesis, it is advisable to perform an amniocentesis.

Diagnosis of fetal anomalies by echography

In this case, echography has a primary role[67]. Certain echographic signs, even though they are non-specific, can alert one to the presence of a fetal infection. These signs include oligohydramnios, an enlarged placenta, hepatosplenomegaly and fetal ascites. In addition, if the fetus also demonstrates a pattern of IUGR, then one can be assured that one is dealing with a fetal infection.

Echography, in addition, gives us information about the possible specific embryonic pathologies, especially in the case of cytomegalovirus, rubella and toxoplasmosis, the three fetal infections that are of greatest risk in IUGR.

In the case of cytomegalovirus, one should be suspicious of this micro-organism in the presence of a clinical episode in the mother that signals this type of infection (e.g. febrile mononucleosis with lymphocytosis, hemolytic anemia, hepatitis with icterus, thrombocytopenia, conjunctivitis, interstitial pneumonia, myocarditis, Guillain–Barré syndrome) or in the case of seroconversion, if the echography demonstrates abnormalities that are clearly associated with this embryonic pathology. Amongst these, in addition to the non-specific abnormalities, we cite intracerebral calcifications (punctiform and periventricular), moderate hydrocephaly (frequently associated with an expansion of the subarachnoid space), microcephaly, intra-abdominal echogenic images, pleural effusions and anasarca.

If the fetal infection is obvious by serological analysis, the echographic evaluation will permit one to define the prognosis by classifying the cases as:

(1) Asymptomatic fetal infection;

(2) Discrete or moderate infection (few echographic findings);

(3) Fetal infection of the pleura and viscera. In this case, which is common in primary infections in the first half of gestation, the perinatal mortality is very high (30–40%) and the risk for perinatal sequelae is very high.

In the case of rubella it is possible to observe various malformations by echography: cardiovascular malformations (patent ductus arteriosis, interventricular defects), anomalies of the central nervous system (microcephaly, cerebral microcalcifications) and hepato-splenomegaly. However, some of the expected abnormalities that have no echographic manifestation (ophthalmic malformations, deafness, mental retardation, immunological abnormalities, behavioral abnormalities) should make us cautious in predicting the prognosis. It should be taken into account that serious abnormalities are the rule before 11 weeks of gestation; in contrast, important abnormalites are rarely found after 18 weeks of gestation.

With respect to toxoplasmosis, the usual case is that the embryonic infection provokes an abortion or 'intrauterine death'. In the fetus, the lesions are essentially cerebral. The ventricular enlargements are usually bilateral and symmetrical, and often originate in the occipital horns. The intracranial calcifications are the consequence of zones of necrotic cerebrum. Other anomalies such as intrahepatic densities, ascites and pericardial effusions are also possible.

The prognosis depends on the gestational age in which the fetal infection occurs and the cerebral lesions that are diagnosed echographically. Infections that occur before 10 weeks of gestation and that have cerebral necrotic lesions should be considered to have a very poor neurological prognosis. In contrast, fetuses that are infected in or beyond the second trimester and that have only isolated calcifications may suffer only from epilepsy and not necessarily from mental retardation. The rapid evolution of the lesions (ventricular dilatation, for example) should also signal a poor prognosis.

FETAL HEMODYNAMICS

The introduction of Doppler has permitted non-invasive evaluation of the flow velocity of various maternal and fetal vessels (Doppler velocimetry)[68–71]. Naturally, this technology is not meant to make the diagnosis of IUGR, as some studies have suggested[72], but rather to predict utero-placental circulatory insufficiency.

For this reason, this technique is especially useful for cases of IUGR that are due to pregnancy-induced hypertension, since this pathological condition is frequently accompanied by vascular changes in the uteroplacental bed or the fetal circulation[73].

In previous studies, our group has published, in addition to standard curves for the indices of flow and resistance in the arcuate and umbilical arteries[74,75], results obtained from given pathologies, such as twin gestation[76], pregnancy-induced hypertension[73,77], diabetes[78] and fetal IUGR[79].

In this chapter, we would like to present our experience regarding the use of Doppler in fetal IUGR, reviewing the capabilities of the technique in studying the uterine, placental and fetal circulation in this pathological process.

Even though quantification by Doppler of

the volume of flow is possible, it is hampered by several important problems, not only because of the distortion that occurs from the lesser or greater angle between the ultrasound wave and the course of the vessel, but also because of the difficulty in determining the section area of the vessel with precision[80]. In spite of the help of color Doppler, the quantification of the volume of flow is a difficult task and is poorly reproducible[81]. For this reason, current practice is to evaluate, by a spectral analysis of flow velocity waveforms (FVW) some vascular resistance indices (RI) that arise from the relationship between the value of the maximum Doppler frequency (Df_{max}) at peak systole (S) and the same value at the lowest point (Df_{min}) at diastole (D). The morphology of the waveform changes according to the resistance that must be overcome by the flow under observation (Figure 9). In order to calculate these indices, it is not necessary to calculate the dimensions of the vessel, and they are independent of the angle of incidence of the ultrasound waves.

The indices that are most used are:

(1) S/D index;

(2) D/S × 100, considered as a vascular 'flow' index, more than a 'resistance' index;

(3) The Pourcelot index[82], calculated by dividing the difference S – D by S;

(4) The pulsatility index S – D/V_m, V_m being the value of the mean velocity throughout the cycle.

The advantage of this last index is that it maintains the proportion of the values regardless of whether the D is negative or reversed.

Uterine circulation

Even though it has been shown that the pathological basis in the development of IUGR can be due to various etiologies, it is clear that one of the most important etiologies is a deficiency of uterine perfusion. An adequate arterial uteroplacental circulation is paramount to assure normal fetal

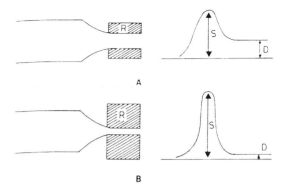

Figure 9 Morphology of the waveform changes according to the resistance (minor (A) or major (B)) that must be overcome by the flow

development during pregnancy. There are an abundance of experimental studies that demonstrate that IUGR is directly related to the progressive increase in uterine flow throughout pregnancy[83], and that a reduction of this flow results in a parallel reduction of fetal growth[84].

Campbell and colleagues[70], Griffin and colleagues[80] and especially Trudinger and colleagues[85,86] have published their experience with Doppler fluxometry in the uterine and arcuate arteries, establishing standard curves of the various indices from the 28th week of gestation until term. In their opinion, this technique enables an accurate study of uteroplacental dynamics and, therefore, of the placental vascular resistance in the maternal sector.

IUGR patterns

Not all fetuses with IUGR reveal abnormal fluxometry indices in the uterine circulation. These are confirmed only in given maternal pathological states such as pregnancy-induced hypertension, especially if they produce secondary ischemic and hemorrhagic lesions in the placenta[87]. However, when the pathological etiology is confined to the fetus, the placenta, or both, without affecting the collateral uterine vasculature, the uterine Doppler findings are normal[88]. For this reason, in approximately 30–40% of cases of

IUGR, such hemodynamic alterations are not confirmed.

Doppler study of the uterine artery has two potential practical applications:

(1) Evaluation of the protodiastolic notch throughout the pregnancy. The persistence of this after 24 weeks of gestation can serve as a screening test for early detection of pregnancies that are at risk for developing IUGR, especially those associated with pre-eclampsia.

(2) Study of the possibility of decreased uterine perfusion in the third trimester, by using the standard curves for each fluxometry index.

Early study of the notch The fact that the anatomic pathological lesions that give rise to the development of IUGR usually appear months before ultrasonographic confirmation of IUGR has led to a search for a high-risk 'marker' capable of identifying possibly affected gravid patients during this uneventful period.

It seems logical to deduce that, as long as the fundamental lesion consists of the absence of the second wave of intravascular colonization of the spiral and radial arteries by the trophoblast, color Doppler examination of the uteroplacental circulation could be a good predictive element. For this reason, Campbell and co-workers[89] as well as Arduini and co-workers[90] have proposed an early Doppler velocimetry study (16–20 weeks of gestation) of the uterine–arcuate arterial system as a risk index for IUGR and pre-eclampsia.

Campbell and associates[89] reported that a Doppler velocimetry study of the uterine circulation, carried out at 16–18 weeks of gestation, was capable of predicting hypertensive pathology and IUGR with a sensitivity of 68% and a specificity of 69%. Currently, Campbell's group proposes that a routine evaluation should be carried out between 18 and 22 weeks, and repeated between 24 and 26 weeks if the protodiastolic notch persists[91].

This procedure has been simplified when one considers that the fundamental prognosticator is the persistence of the notch after 24 weeks, and not necessarily the value of the different indices. The persistence of the notch after this time[92,93] portends a poor prognosis[94].

If the evolution of a hypertensive state of pregnancy is detected early by Doppler study of the uteroplacental flow, a considerable value is gained, given the possibility of primary prevention of this risk with small doses of acetylsalicylic acid (1 mg/kg per day), as suggested by several authors[95–98].

The large number of false positives and the poor positive predictive value that this procedure entails are probably explained by the biochemical and hemodynamic compensatory mechanisms that occur in the second half of pregnancy[99]. This is also why certain authors[100] feel that this procedure should not be introduced as a routine screening test in nulliparous women, even though these findings are associated with an increased risk for pre-eclampsia and IUGR.

Advanced or late study of Doppler velocimetry Jacobson and associates[101] carried out a study of uteroplacental velocimetry in 93 gravid women with supposed IUGR between 20 and 24 weeks of gestation, observing a statistically significant association between the indices of resistance that were abnormally high at this time, and confirming IUGR after delivery. As observed in Table 5 a reasonable sensitivity (70%) was achieved, with a specificity of 64% but a very low positive predictive value (33%). Given this fact, the authors deduced that the great number of false positives limited the clinical value of these observations.

On the other hand, Bruinse and co-workers[102] found only a 16.9% sensitivity and a 10% positive predictive value, even when the specificity and negative predictive value were high (95.1% and 79.6%, respectively), in a group of patients at 28 weeks of gestation whose newborns were small for gestational age.

If these studies are carried out later, in the final trimester of gestation, the figures for the positive predictive value clearly improve, and

Table 5 Advanced study of uteroplacental velocimetry

Year	Author	Week	n	IUGR (%)	Sensitivity (%)	Specificity (%)	PPV (%)	NPV (%)
1989	Bruinse et al.[102]	28	405	22	16.9	95.1	10.0	79.6
1990	Jacobson et al.[101]	20–24	93	18	70.0	64.0	33.0	89.0

PPV, positive predictive value; NPV, negative predictive value; IUGR, intrauterine growth restriction

Table 6 Uterine flow and type of intrauterine growth restriction (IUGR)

IUGR type	Cases	Pathological uterine flow
IUGR I	28	1 (3.57%)
IUGR II	37	22 (59.45%)
IUGR III	15	2 (13.33%)
Non-classifiable IUGR	9	3 (33.33%)
Total	89	28 (31.46%)

were situated at 53%[85,102] and 66%[103], but consequently, the figures for sensitivity decreased to between 22%[102] and 60%[85]. Some authors contend that uterine Doppler examination should be introduced in the second trimester in all gravid patients as a screening test for IUGR and pre-eclampsia[104].

Using pulsed Doppler, we studied 89 gravid patients between 30 and 40 weeks of gestation carrying fetuses subjected to severe IUGR that was later confirmed at delivery. The cases were classified according to our criteria[105]. The results are shown in Table 6.

Umbilical circulation

An adequate blood flow through the umbilical vessels is essential for adequate nutrition and oxygenation of the fetus. Therefore, the quantification of this flow makes it possible to study, in an objective manner, the efficiency of the placental circulation and, in general, fetal well-being. It is especially useful in cases of high risk and suspicion or evidence of IUGR.

In both pulsed and continuous Doppler, one obtains FVW values of notable pulsatility and low Df telediastole, which translates into considerable vascular resistance that exists in the fetal sector of the placenta, the opposite of which occurs in the maternal sector, and in spite of the presence of a minimum vascular tone in the umbilical arteries.

From the physiological point of view, the resistance indices measure the difficulty that the column of blood faces as it advances through the umbilical artery to the placenta to perfuse the intricate arterial network in the fetal sector of the organ. These resistances, notably greater than in the maternal sector, diminish as the gestation progresses. In practice, this is due to the gradual increase in velocities at the end of pregnancy.

IUGR patterns

Morrow and colleagues[106], working with fetal lambs subjected to an embolization of the capillary microcirculation (by means of plastic microemboli measuring 50 μm in diameter), observed gradual changes in the FVW of the umbilical artery similar to those that have been described in human fetuses subjected to IUGR due to capillary pathology (reduced diastolic flow, zero diastole, and finally reverse flow).

The reason for this deterioration in the FVW resides in the increase of the vascular resistance at the level of the placental microcirculation, which, by the time it induces a perfusional deficit in the umbilical artery, causes a progressive decrease in the po_2 of the umbilical vein due to an inadequate exchange of gas at the capillary level.

Hypoxemia, therefore, is the consequence and not the cause of the hemodynamic alterations that occur in the placental microcirculation and the umbilical artery. Effectively, a reduction in the po_2 without a placental lesion does not cause a change in the umbilical FVW[107–109], neither does an increase in the hematic viscosity or an increase in the maternal arterial blood pressure[110].

In humans, it appears clear that the placental lesion consists not only of obvious structural changes[111], but also of a significant reduction in the number of arterioles in the tertiary chorionic villi[112], up to the point that an inverse relationship is established between the S/D ratio and the number of these arterioles[113]. This reduction in tertiary arterioles is due to several causes: the lack of their formation by interference in the maturation of the placenta, obliteration by thrombotic and coagulation phenomena and, in many cases, the reduction of the uteroplacental perfusion that induces a hypoxic ischemia of the intervillus space and vasoconstriction of the villous arterioles[114]. Jackson and colleagues[115] have shown, by means of stereological placental studies, that there are statistically significant differences in the surface and volume of the villus arterioles in placentas of newborns that are small or appropriate for gestational age, and this fact obviously influences the pulsatility index of the umbilical artery.

The reduction, whether functional or organic, of the number of arterioles in the tertiary villi due to a pathological process inherent to the placenta, or, in contrast, the presence of circulatory difficulties in the fetus that cause a reduction in the blood supply, or both processes together, can significantly alter the character of the FVW in the umbilical artery. In addition, one cannot exclude an increase in viscosity of the blood or a reduction in the arterial pressure.

An increase in the resistance index (or the decrease in flow) that falls below the limits of confidence of standard curves should alert one to the possible deterioration of the fetal condition. This suspicion is reinforced if the diastolic flow becomes minimal or non-existent, or especially if there is reverse flow. There are four possible stages within the spectrum of pathological patterns[116,117]:

Stage I The velocities of the diastolic component of the FVW are below normal values, which results in an alteration of the mentioned indices of resistance and flow.

Nevertheless, in spite of the described placental morphological findings, the indices of resistance or pulsatility in the villous arteries identified by color Doppler and evaluated by pulsed Doppler are apparently normal[118] in IUGR, contrasting with the umbilical indices in these same patients which are clearly altered. Besides the fact that color Doppler probably selects those vessels that have better blood flow, it can be argued that the arterioles that remain intact attempt to compensate for the overall reduction in their number by having a normal or increased blood flow. The inability to detect intraplacental color Doppler signals portends a grave prognosis in this pathology.

This pattern is the one frequently observed in fetuses with IUGR that do not manifest fetal hypoxia[119].

Stage II End-diastolic flow is missing. The value of telediastole is zero. This finding appears to correlate with the initiation of the centralization of flow.

Stage III No flow is observed throughout diastole. This pattern is usually associated with grave fetal hypoxia, which often manifests as abnormal fetal heart rate patterns.

Stage IV A reverse or inverse flow in diastole is confirmed[120]. Severe fetal hypoxia normally exists in this stage. The fetus is at serious risk for intrauterine fetal demise. Abnormal umbilical indices are consistently associated with IUGR with a sensitivity of 40–50% and a specificity of more than 90%.

When the absence of diastolic flow is recorded, or in the presence of reverse flow, these pregnancies normally have an abnormal evolution, and perinatal results are poor[119,121–127]. When one compares IUGR fetuses with equal severity but with or without these Doppler findings, fetal deaths occur more commonly in the first group[119,122,128]. In addition, the literature insists that fetuses with IUGR that have absent or reverse flow in telediastole present not only a high fetal and neonatal mortality rate, but also a greater incidence of permanent neurological damage[126]. The value of these findings is also evident in twin gestations with ponderal discordancy[129].

In recent years, several authors[130–132] have supported the utility of the registering the FVW of the umbilical artery in all gestations at risk, but especially in those that demonstrate or are at risk for IUGR[72,86,120,133]. Moreover, this can be achieved using low-cost continuous Doppler equipment[134].

To establish the prognosis of IUGR, some authors[134] have suggested the introduction of special indices such as the compliance–weight deficit index (CWDI) that combines the deficit in the compliance of the umbilical artery with the deficit in weight using established specific linear regressions. In our opinion, the complexity of this procedure makes it difficult to incorporate it into clinical practice.

In our study that has already been mentioned using 82 gravid patients with various types of IUGR, all patients with type I IUGR had normal umbilical artery indices (100%). In type II, on the other hand, 51.35% of patients manifested pathological indices, the percentage diminishing to 13.33% in those patients with type III IUGR. The contribution of real-time Doppler consists of its capability to establish the type of IUGR[77, 135].

As is well known, there are three types of IUGR: type I (harmonious and precocious), the origin being an intrinsic reduction in potential growth; type II (asymmetric and late in onset), owing to a vascular uteroplacental insufficiency; and type III, or mixed.

In type I, genetically small but without chromosomal aberrations, the velocimetric indices of the uterine and umbilical arteries are normal[134]. In contrast, if a genetic abnormality exists, even though the uterine indices will be normal, the umbilical indices will be pathological.

In type II, where a placental insufficiency exists, the velocimetric indices are first altered in the uterine arteries (very early in onset if there is pre-eclampsia), and subsequently in the umbilical arteries. For this reason, a high proportion of pathological indices are observed in addition to indices that are at the limits of normality, not only in the uterine artery but also in the umbilical artery.

In type III, the proportion of abnormal results, in both the uterine and the umbilical arteries, is low.

Several authors have attempted to predict intrapartum fetal distress in fetuses with IUGR by using color Doppler during pregnancy. Rochelson and co-workers[119] confirmed the presence of fetal distress in 53% of cases with IUGR with pathological umbilical indices, and Brar and Platt[121] raised this figure to 75% in cases of FVW without telediastolic flow or reversed flow.

Fetal circulation

It is possible to observe and characterize the majority of fetal vessels with color-coded Doppler, and, with continuous or pulsed Doppler, it is possible to obtain the flow FVW. The FVW can be analyzed by using indices in a qualitative or semi-quantitative fashion to acertain the volume of flow.

Fetal arterial circulation: IUGR patterns

Fetal descending aorta An important percentage of fetuses subjected to IUGR with progressive diminution of the po_2 in the umbilical vein, demonstrate a secondary reduction in the telediastolic FVW of the aorta that eventually leads to the complete absence or even reversal of the flow[123,136].

This process is basically the same as that which we have already described for the umbilical artery. However, important differences exist that explain not only the different timing of these changes, but also their pathophysiological significance.

The increase in the umbilical pusatility index is caused, as we have already seen, by placental lesions that increase the resistance at this level. This local factor acts secondarily and at a later date to influence the aortic pulsatility index. In contrast, this is not only subjected to the possible increase in flow of the aortic branches (40% of the uterine flow is diverted to the placenta), but also to the cardiac compensatory mechanisms that, for a given time, will work to prevent alteration of the aortic pulsatility index. Herein lies the explanation of the fact that the umbilical artery pulsatility index is usually first affected, and only subsequently the aortic pulsatility index.

These changes in the aortic FVW usually precede cardiotocographic abnormalities by 3 days[116,137], even though, on some occasions, this time interval can be measured in weeks.

As we discuss further on, there is a statistically significant relationship between the degree of fetal hypoxia, measured by cordocentesis, and the type of FVW and its median velocity[138,139] in the aorta. However, no significant relationship has been demonstrated between the Doppler findings and the fetal metabolic state.

Several authors have established the predictive capacity of the aortic FVW of the morbidity and mortality of the fetus, especially in cases of IUGR. Laurin and colleagues[116] have demonstrated that the aortic pulsatility index is capable of predicting 63% of fetuses that develop fetal distress during labor, and this figure is increased to 87% if the FVW is classified according to the class system. Hackett and associates[140] have observed that the absence of diastolic values in the aorta predicts neonatal morbidity in a significant manner. This finding, and especially in the presence of reverse flow, is associated with a very high incidence of neonatal complications, especially necrotizing enterocolitis, which is not observed in fetuses with the same degree of IUGR but without Doppler changes of the aortic artery. Marsal and associates[141] have correlated the results from Doppler studies of the fetal aorta (FVW with or without telediastolic values) with neonatal morbidity.

The accumulated evidence suggests that monitoring of the aortic FVW is a good secondary test to evaluate the well-being of fetuses that appear on ultrasound examination to be growing poorly[142].

Fetal renal artery   Animal models suggest that increased cerebral perfusion occurs at the expense of the perfusion of certain organs, such as the kidney.

Vyas and co-workers[143,144] have attempted to correlate the degree of fetal hypoxemia in umbilical vessels with the pulsatility index of the renal artery in a group of fetuses with IUGR. The conclusion was that the pulsatility index of the renal artery was indeed greater than the median pulsatility index in a normal group of fetuses in a significant number of cases. In contrast, a significant relationship could not be demonstrated between the change in pulsatility index (ΔPI) and the change in po_2 (Δpo_2). Nevertheless, if fetuses less than 24 weeks of gestation are excluded, this association is clearly demonstrated ($p > 0.05$; $r = -0.368$; constant = 1.515; slope = 0.424; DE residual = 1.381). These findings suggest that the vascular response to hypoxemia occurs only if the organ is sufficiently mature.

As is well known, prolonged hypoxemia in some organs such as the intestine or liver can lead to serious neonatal complications such as necrotizing enterocolitis and hemorrhage. Currently, we are not able easily to evaluate the FVW of arteries that supply these organs, but it is possible that the study of the renal arteries, facilitated by color Doppler, could be representative of the visceral perfusion as a whole. Hackett and colleagues[140] observed that when there was an absence of diastolic values in the FVW of the aorta and the renal arteries, there was an increase in the stated complications, and there was a direct relationship between the pulsatility index and the severity of the hypoxemia[143]. On the other hand, there is an inverse relationship between the pulsatility index and the amniotic fluid volume[145]. This suggests that the pulsatility index of the renal artery can be considered as a good marker for renal perfusion and is thus useful in controlling fetal adaptation to hypoxemia[88].

Fetal common carotid artery The values of the diastolic frequencies increase as the umbilical pO_2 decreases, but with a definite delay compared to the intracranial findings.

Bilardo and associates[146], in addition to observing a gradual reduction in the pulsatility indices, confirmed a good correlation between the pulsatility index and the mean velocity in the aorta with data from the acid–base equilibrium obtained from cordocentesis. A significant correlation was noted between the reduction in the pulsatility index and the FVW of the common carotid artery and the degree of hypoxia and acidemia.

Fetal cerebral vessels Wladimiroff and co-workers[147] were the first to describe the use of Doppler to obtain the FVW of the intracranial vessels (internal carotid artery, cerebral arteries). More recently, Van den Wijngaard and associates[148] carried out a study of these vessels. In all of the cases, an increase in the value of the diastolic frequencies was noted, indicating a reduction in the resistance at this level, as a response to a vasomotor (vasodilatation) effect. Other authors[149] have reported similar conclusions and observed a fall in the resistance index in 28% of cases with IUGR. Apparently, the fall in cerebral vascular resistance is associated with an increase in hypoxic encephalopathy in the neonate[150].

The comparison between the pulsatility index of the median cerebral artery and the pO_2, pCO_2 and pH in fetal blood obtained by cordocentesis demonstrates a significant correlation between the two parameters[146,151]. Nevertheless, this relationship does not appear to be close enough to deduce that the cerebral pulsatility index can be used to quantify the acid–base status of the fetus, and

make decisions about the optimal timing of the delivery[88].

Intracardiac circulation: IUGR patterns
Cardiovascular hemodynamic changes occurring in fetuses with placental insufficiency can be summarized as follows. The 'brain-sparing effect' in response to hypoxemia causes cardiac hemodynamic changes with decreased left ventricle afterload due to cerebral vasodilatation and increased right ventricle afterload due to systemic vasoconstriction. Furthermore, hypoxemia impairs myocardial contractility, and polycythemia alters blood viscosity and therefore preload[152]. As a consequence, fetuses with IUGR show impaired ventricular filling expressed by an increase in the early and active ventricular filling ratio in both ventricles[153,154], as well as decreased aortic and pulmonary artery blood flow (more evident in the pulmonary artery)[155–157] and increased and decreased time to peak velocities in the aortic and pulmonary valves, respectively, in response to changes of ventricular afterload[158]. Finally, there is an increase in left cardiac output in relation to right cardiac output[156,159]. In short, these hemodynamic intracardiac changes are compatible with a preferential shift of cardiac output in favor of the left ventricle, leading to improved perfusion of the brain.

A detailed review of the sequence of intracardiac hemodynamic changes in association with placental insufficiency is presented in this chapter. In fetal life, both ventricles work in parallel, providing blood perfusion to two vascular systems that are connected by physiological shunts. As a result of hemodynamic changes occurring in the circulation of the fetus, both preload and afterload of the right and left ventricles can be compromised, resulting in different adaptive responses, given the particular anatomical and functional characteristics of each ventricle[160,161].

Afterload ventricular changes of the left ventricle The upper half of the fetal body is perfused by 70% of the left ventricle afterload. In cases of placental insufficiency, hypoxemia, hypercapnia and metabolic acidosis cause cerebral and coronary vasodilatation which results in decreased left ventricle afterload[162,163].

Afterload ventricular changes of the right ventricle   Ninety per cent of the right ventricle afterload flows through the thoracic duct to the fetal descending aorta and, for this reason, this parameter is influenced by changes in the vascular resistance of peripheral territories. Among these, the umbilical territory plays a major role, owing to its high volume and low resistance. In cases of placental insufficiency, increased peripheral resistance causes a significant increase in right ventricle afterload, a main differential characteristic between fetuses affected by symmetrical or asymmetrical IUGR. Despite this increase in the peripheral resistance, it has been shown that pressure in the descending aorta is maintained, probably attributable to a decrease in the right ventricle cardiac output[164].

Balance between the two vascular systems   According to opposite ventricular afterload changes in cases of placental insufficiency (decrease in the left ventricle and increase in the right ventricle), the sensitivity of Doppler velocimetry indices that relate the cerebral and umbilical circulations is higher than that provided by the measurement of each individual index[165]. Furthermore, the isthmus of the aorta, the only arterial connecting passage of the two vascular systems, is particularly sensitive to hemodynamic changes occurring in the cerebral and/or placental territory. A constant diastolic flow is usually detected at this level, owing to the low placental resistance[166]. In cases of placental insufficiency, experimental[164] and clinical[167] studies have demonstrated an increased resistance at this level with reverse diastolic flow, probably preceding changes documented in the umbilical circulation[168]. As vascular resistance increases, blood flow

through the aortic isthmus may become insignificant, leading to complete separation of the two vascular systems[169].

Preload ventricular changes   Preload ventricular function is clinically assessed by measuring ventricular pressure or end-diastolic volume. Clinical study of factors involved in ventricular preload is complex. Although both ventricles perfuse two parallel vascular systems, the venous blood return of each system does not follow a parallel pattern. In fact, the left ventricle preload is mainly determined by the size of the oval foramen and the blood flow from the inferior vena cava, and to a lesser extent by pulmonary blood flow. On the other hand, the right ventricle preload is mainly related to blood flow from the superior vena cava and the percentage of flow from the inferior vena cava that is directly derived to the right ventricular chamber.

Preload changes of the left ventricle   Increased impedance in the placental territory is followed by increased umbilical resistance and a reduction of blood flow at this level, which determines a decrease in the venous return from the inferior vena cava, with reduction in the blood supply to both ventricles. Despite the involvement of both cavities, data from experimental[161,170] and clinical[156,159] studies indicate a greater involvement of the right ventricle than the left ventricle, attributable to the increase in the percentage of blood flow from the inferior vena cava derived through the oval foramen and/or to the increase in pulmonary venous return (secondary to the increased pressure in the descending aorta and the pulmonary artery). This last phenomenon would account for the incidence of persistent pulmonary hypertension in newborns with asymmetrical IUGR[171,172]. In turn, the myocardial response to preload and afterload changes is different in both ventricles, determining different ventricular adaptive responses in situations of hemodynamic compromise, which finally results in a better response of the right ventricle, leading to maintenance of near-normal levels of perfusion to the brain.

Preload changes of the right ventricle In cases of placental insufficiency, right ventricle preload is preserved, because of opposite hemodynamic changes in the venous return, with a decrease in the blood flow from the inferior vena cava and an increase in the blood flow from the superior vena cava (secondary to cerebral vasodilatation)[161].

Myocardial function changes Myocardial function can be affected by changes in ventricular preload and afterload due to factors such as chronic hypoxemia, acidosis or a decrease in essential amino acids. Histopathological studies have shown intrinsic myocardial lesions in fetuses with severe IUGR[173], which may be expressed in either systolic or diastolic functions. In M-mode ultrasound studies, myocardial function impairment is preferentially documented by a decrease in the right ventricle shortening fraction with an increase in the relationship of the end-diastolic diameter between the right and the left ventricles[174]. Doppler velocimetry reveals a decrease in maximal velocimetry waveforms in the descending aorta and pulmonary artery[156,157,159] and a reduction of the acceleration time in the pulmonary artery[158].

Changes in diastolic myocardial function The pattern of ventricular diastolic flow studied by means of Doppler ultrasonography of the atrioventricular valves corresponds to the E velocity waveform of early ventricular filling and the A velocity waveform of end-diastolic atrial contraction. In normal conditions and during intrauterine life, the A velocity waveform predominates over the E waveform, owing to the low compliance of the fetal myocardium, although there is a progressive increase of the E/A ratio by improvement as gestation progresses[175]. Fetuses with asymmetrical IUGR show a characteristic increase of the E/A ratio as compared with controls of the same gestational age (secondary to afterload changes)[153,154], an increase of deceleration time of the E waveform (indicating a difficulty in ventricular relaxation)[176,177] and an increase in the percentage of reverse flow of the inferior vena cava (secondary to decreased myocardial compliance)[175,178].

Changes in systolic myocardial function In these situations of fetal hemodynamic compromise, there is a reduction of cardiac output in both ventricles (higher on the right side)[170] that is proportional to duration of the insult[156,159]. These differences in the degree of impairment of ventricular function can be related to the distinctive morphology of both chambers and/or differences in aortic and pulmonary artery impedances[179]. On the other hand, there may be an increase in the cardiothoracic index, which may be secondary to a myocardial lesion due to hypoxemia or polycythemia, or to a reduction of the thoracic circumference secondary to fetal growth impairment[180].

Fetal venous circulation: IUGR patterns

In vivo study of the fetal venous circulation is more difficult, except for the umbilical vein, owing to problems in the correct identification of vessels and to the complexity in the morphological interpretation of velocimetry waveforms. The ductus venosus and the inferior vena cava, owing to its proximity to the heart, are the vessels in which a direct relationship between pressure and flow throughout the cardiac cycle is more reliably reflected. The application of Doppler ultrasonography to the assessment of fetal blood flow has been extended to the venous circulation over past years, and this is a promising field for improving our knowledge of fetal hemodynamics.

The ductus venosus is the main structure for distributing oxygenated blood to fetal tissues in intrauterine life[181]. Its geometrical characteristics (small-caliber vessel) and its anatomical position (unique direct communication between the umbilical vein and the right atrium) provide the capacity for regulating oxygenated blood in situations of hemodynamic compromise. Accordingly, in the presence of hypoxemia, a preferential passage of blood flow from the umbilical vein to the ductus venosus takes place, with subsequent reduction of the intrahepatic circulation[182,183]. In addition, it seems that there is an active intrinsic mechanism at this level, which would be able to induce blood flow modifications. Endings of the celiac plexus, phrenic nerve and vagus nerve in the muscular thickness of its wall have been reported, so that the ductus venosus may act as a sphincter regulated by the sympathetic and parasympathetic autonomic nervous system[182]. Moreover, local factors, such as prostaglandins, responsible for maintaining ductal patency would also act at this level. Despite its main role as oxygenated blood supplier in cases of hemodynamic impairment, other compensatory mechanisms should be present, given that occlusion of the ductus venosus in experimental animals is not followed by measurable changes of oxygen saturation in the aortic and carotid vessels[183]. Although it is not an essential structure, occlusion or absence of the ductus venosus would determine a lower capacity to cope with placental impairment[183,184]. The ductus venosus shows a characteristic triphasic velocimetry waveform, with a peak of maximal velocity at ventricular systole, a second peak during initiation of diastole and a minimal velocity in the end-diastolic period, coinciding with atrial contraction[185,186]. In fetuses with IUGR, although maximal velocity is maintained, there is a reduction of end-diastolic velocity even up to a reverse of flow[187]. This may be secondary to the increased end-diastolic volume in response to an increase in peripheral resistances and a reduction of the myocardial response capacity, when compensatory mechanisms are surpassed and there is a reduction of blood flow supply to the cardiac muscle[188].

In normal conditions of intrauterine life, the inferior vena cava shows a triphasic flow pattern corresponding to ventricular systole, the early diastolic phase and the late diastolic phase (atrial contraction). The first two waveforms are positive and the third is reversed. The percentage of reverse flow coinciding with atrial contraction reflects the end-diastolic pressure gradient between the right atrium and the right ventricle, and decreases progressively with advancing gestation, so that in normal conditions it exceeds 10% of the total flow[181]. This reveals the improvement of ventricular compliance and the reduction of right ventricular afterload due to a physiological fall of impedance in the uteroplacental vascular territory. Fetuses with IUGR showed, at this level, an increase of reverse flow coinciding with atrial contraction, which may have reached up to 30%[175,178,182].

In normal pregnancies, umbilical venous blood flow is usually continuous, although before the 12th week of gestation synchronous pulsations with heart rate reflecting the stiffness of myocardial fibers at this early gestational age may be present[189,190]. From the second trimester of pregnancy, their presence indicates myocardial impairment, and has a significance similar to that of increased reverse flow in the inferior vena cava. In fact, in fetuses with IUGR, the presence of pulsations in the umbilical vein has been significantly associated with an increase in perinatal mortality[191,192].

Fetal hemodynamic profile

Thanks to the efforts of various investigators[139,140,144,146,151,193] we can depend on standard curves of the FVW (median velocity and velocimetric indices) of the principal fetal vessels: the umbilical artery and veins, the aorta, the common and internal carotid arteries, the cerebral arteries (anterior, median and posterior), the renal artery, the iliac arteries and the hypogastric arteries.

Currently, with the use of centile curves of the pulsatility index with discriminative values for each week of gestation, better quantification of the obtained data has been possible. By using standard curves of normality, we have been able to design a 'hemodynamic profile' that is much more precise and adapted to each week of pregnancy (Table 7). However, it is important

Table 7 Hemodynamic profile. Pulsatility indices

	Normal	*Abnormal*
Umbilical artery	< 95th centile	> 95th centile
Thoracic aorta	< 95th centile	> 95th centile
Common carotid artery	> 5th centile	< 5th centile
Middle cerebral artery	> 5th centile	< 5th centile

to remember that all of the cerebral arteries normally show a significant drop in the pulsatility index in the final 7–8 weeks of gestation. According to Hudlicka and Tyler[194], this is attributable to a certain degree of 'physiological cerebral preservation' resulting from the gradual decrease of the fetal po_2 and to a maturation process of arteriolar proliferation. This phenomenon needs to be kept in mind so as that errors in interpreting the data are not committed.

On the other hand, this new focal point has permitted meticulous study of the different stages of the pathological redistribution of flow. These types of studies require not only adequate equipment (pulsed Doppler machine (duplex system) with a sectorial ultrasound capability and good definition, and supplemented by color Doppler) but also significant experience of the operator. With these requirements met, carrying out a fetal hemodynamic profile is possible in 90% of cases[144,148].

Of all of these possible indices (S/D ratio, resistance index, flow index, etc.) the pulsatility index was chosen as the most useful for the hemodynamic profile.

References

1. Carrera JM, Mallafré J, Krauel J. Organización de una Unidad de Riesgo Fetal Elevado. In *Clínica Ginecológica: Estudio prenatal de la Unidad Feto-Placentaria*, Vol. 2. Barcelona: Salvat, 1977: 1–23
2. Carrera JM, Palombo H. Valoración prenatal del riesgo de crecimiento intrauterino retardado. *Prog Obstet Ginecol* 1978;21:311–18
3. Carrera JM, Alegre M, Mallafré J, *et al.* Aspectos obstétricos del crecimiento intrauterino retardado. Book of Abstracts of the *IV Reunión Nacional de Medicina Perinatal*, Zaragoza, 1982: 239–66
4. Carrera JM, Barri PN. Diagnosis of the intrauterine growth retardation. In Salvadori B, Bacchi-Modena A, eds. *Poor Intrauterine Fetal Growth*. Parma: Minerva Medica, 1977:278
5. Campbell S, Pearce JMF, Hackett G, Cohen-Overbeek T, Hernández C. Quality assessment of uteroplacental blood flow early screening test for high-risk pregnancies. *Obstet Gynecol* 1986;68: 649–53
6. Steele SA, Pearce JM, Chamberlain GV. Doppler ultrasound of the uteroplacental circulation as a screening test for severe preeclampsia with intrauterine growth retardation. *J Obstet Gynecol Reprod Biol* 1988;28:279–87
7. Jacobson SL, Imhof R, Manning N, *et al.* The value of Doppler assessment of the uteroplacental circulation in prediction of preeclampsia or intrauterine growth retardation. *Am J Obstet Gynecol* 1988;162:110–14
8. Westin B. Gravidogram and fetal growth. Comparison with biochemical supervision. *Acta Obstet Gynecol Scand* 1977;56(Suppl):273–82
9. Westin B. Gravidogram and poor intrauterine fetal growth. In Salvadori B, Bacchi-Modena A, eds. *Poor Intrauterine Fetal Growth*. Parma: Minerva Medica, 1977:44–9
10. Effer SB. Management of high-risk pregnancy: a report of a combined obstetrical and neonatal intensive care unit. *Can Med Assoc J* 1969;101:55–63
11. Campbell S, Soothill P. Detection and management of intrauterine growth retardation. A British approach. In Chevernak FA, Isaacson J, Campbell S, eds. *Ultrasound in Obstetrics and Gynecology*. London: Little Brown, 1993:1431

12. Theron GB, Pattinsor RC. Management of patients with poor symphysis pubis–fundus growth by Doppler flow velocimetry of the umbilical artery – an effective method to detect the fetus at risk. *Int J Gynecol Obstet* 1992;39:93–8

13. Pearce JM, Campbell S. A comparison of symphysis–fundal height and ultrasound as screening tests for light for gestational age infants. *Br J Obstet Gynaecol* 1987;94:100–4

14. Goldstein I, Reece EA, Pilu G, Bovicelli L, Hobbins JC. Cerebellar measurements with ultrasonography in the evaluation of fetal growth and development. *Am J Obstet Gynecol* 1987;156: 1065–9

15. Reece EA, Godstein I, Pilu G, Hobbins JC. Fetal cerebellar growth unaffected by intrauterine growth retardation: a new parameter for prenatal diagnosis. *Am J Obstet Gynecol* 1987;157:632–8

16. Reece EA, Hagay Z. Prenatal diagnosis of deviant fetal growth. In Reece AE, Hobbins JC, Mahoney MJ, Petrie RH, eds. *Medicine of the Fetus and Mother*. Philadelphia: Lippincot, 1992:671–85

17. Duchatel F, Mennesson B, Berseneff H, Oury JF. Antenatal echographic measurement of the fetal cerebellum. Significance in the evaluation of fetal development. *J Gynecol Obstet Biol Reprod Paris* 1989;18:879–83

18. Campbell WA, Narci D, Vintzileos AM, Rodis JF, Turner CW, Egan JF. Transverse cerebellar diameter/abdominal circumference ratio throughout pregnancy: a gestational age independent method to assess fetal growth. *Obstet Gynecol* 1991;77:893–96

19. Drumm JE, Clinch J, MacKenzie G. The ultrasonic measurement of fetal crown–rump length as a method of assessing gestational age. *Br J Obstet Gynaecol* 1976;83:417–21

20. Shepard M, Filly RA. A standardized plane for biparietal diameter measurement. *J Ultrasound Med* 1982;1:145–54

21. Johnson ML, Dunne MG, Mack LA, Rashbaum CL. Evaluation of fetal intracranial anatomy by static and real-time ultrasound. *J Clin Ultrasound* 1980;8:311–18

22. Campbell S. Ultrasonic fetal cephalometry during the second trimester of pregnancy. *J Obstet Gynaecol Br Commonw* 1970;77:1057–63

23. Varma YR. Prediction of delivery date by ultrasound cephalometry. *Br J Obstet Gynaecol* 1973;80:316–19

24. Campbell S, Newman GB. Growth of the fetal biparietal diameter during normal pregnancy. *J Obstet Gynaecol Br Commonw* 1971;78:513–19

25. Campbell S, Dewhurst CJ. Diagnosis of the small for date fetus by serial ultrasonic cephalometry. *Lancet* 1971;2:1002–6

26. Seeds JW. Impaired fetal growth: ultrasonic evaluation and clinical management. *Obstet Gynecol* 1984;63:577–82

27. Rosendahl H, Kivinen S. Routine ultrasound screening for early detection of small for gestational age fetuses. *Obstet Gynecol* 1988;71: 518–21

28. Arias F. The diagnosis and management of intrauterine growth retardation. *Obstet Gynecol* 1977;49:293–8

29. Kurjak A, Kirkinen P, Latin V. Biometric and dynamic ultrasound assessment of small-for-dates infants. Report of 260 cases. *Obstet Gynecol* 1980;56:281–4

30. Geirsson RT, Patel NB, Christie AD. Intrauterine volume, fetal abdominal area and biparietal diameter measurements with ultrasound in the prediction of small-for-dates babies in a high-risk obstetric population. *Br J Obstet Gynaecol* 1985;92:936–40

31. Sabbagha R, Hughey M, Depp R. Growth adjusted sonographic age. A simplified method. *Obstet Gynecol* 1978;51:383–6

32. Campbell S, Newman GB. Growth of the fetal biparietal diameter during normal pregnancy. *Br J Obstet Gynaecol* 1971;75:513–19

33. Macler J, Rosenthal C, Burgun P, Renaud R. The interest of ecography measurements of the transversal abdominal diameter in the poor intrauterine fetal growth. In Salvadori B, Bacchi-Modena A, eds. *Poor Intrauterine Fetal Growth.* Parma: Minerva Medica, 1977

34. Zoltan I. Poor intrauterine fetal growth: constitutional factors/weight and size. In Salvadori B, Bacchi-Modena A, eds. *Poor Intrauterine Fetal Growth.* Parma: Minerva Medica, 1977:51–5

35. Campbell S, Wilkin D. Ultrasonic measurement of fetal abdomen circumference in the estimation of fetal weight. *Br J Obstet Gynaecol* 1975;82:689–97

36. Jeanty P, Coussaert E, Contraine F. Normal growth of the abdominal perimeter. *Am J Perinatol* 1984;1:129–35

37. Wittmann BK, Robinson HP, Aitchison T, Fleming JE. The value of diagnostic ultrasound as a screening test for intrauterine growth retardation: comparison of nine parameters. *Am J Obstet Gynecol* 1979;134:30–5

38. Carrera JM, Alegre M, Torrents M. Ecobiometría anatómica fetal. In Carrera JM, ed. *Ecografía Obstétrica*. Barcelona: Salvat, 1985:259–86

39. Warsof SL, Cooper DJ, Little D, Campbell S. Routine ultrasound screening for antenatal detection of intrauterine growth retardation. *Obstet Gynecol* 1986;67:33–9

40. Warsof SL, Wolf P, Coulehan J, Queenan JT. Comparison of fetal weight estimation formulas with and without head measurements. *Obstet Gynecol* 1986;67:569–73

41. Campbell S, Thoms A. Ultrasound measurement of the fetal head to abdomen circumference ratio in the assessment of growth retardation. *Br J Obstet Gynaecol* 1977;84:165–74

42. O'Brien GD, Queenan JT. Growth of the ultrasound fetal femur length during normal pregnancy. *Am J Obstet Gynecol* 1981;141:833–7

43. O'Brien GD, Queenan JT. Ultrasound femur length in relation to intrauterine growth retardation. *Am J Obstet Gynecol* 1982;144:35–9

44. Hadlock FP, Deter RL, Harrist RB, Roecker E, Park SK. A date independent predictor of intrauterine growth retardation: femur length/abdominal circumference ratio. *Am J Roentgenol* 1983;141:979–84

45. Benson CB, Doubilet PM, Saltzman DH, Jones TB. FL/AC ratio: poor predictor of intrauterine growth retardation. *Invest Radiol* 1985;20:727–30

46. Japanese Society of Obstetrics and Gynecology. Standard ultrasonic values of biparietal diameter and femur length of Japanese fetuses. *Acta Obstet Gynecol Jpn* 1993;45:391–4

47. Gohari P, Berkowitz RL, Hobbins JC. *In utero* prediction of IUGR by determination of total intrauterine volume. *Am J Obstet Gynecol* 1977;127: 255–8

48. Hata T, Deter RL. A review of fetal organ measurements obtained with ultrasound: normal growth. *J Clin Ultrasound* 1992;20:155–74

49. Campbell S, Silkin D. Ultrasonic measurement of fetal abdominal circumference in estimation of fetal weight. *Br J Obstet Gynaecol* 1975;82: 689

50. Hadlock FP, Harrist RB, Sherman RS, *et al.* Estimation of fetal weight with the use of head, body and femur measurements. *Am J Obstet Gynecol* 1985;151:333–7

51. Shepard MJ, Richards VA, Berkowitz RL, *et al.* An evaluation of two equations for predicting fetal weight using ultrasound measurements. *Am J Obstet Gynecol* 1982;142:47–54

52. Rose B, MacCallum WD. A simplified method for estimating fetal weight using ultrasound measurements. *Obstet Gynecol* 1987;69:671

53. Aoki M, Ogata M. Ultrasonic diagnosis of IUGR. *Shusanki Igaku* 1982;12:419

54. Shinozuka N. Formulas for fetal weight estimation by ultrasound measurements based on neonatal specific gravities and volume. *Am J Obstet Gynecol* 1987;157:1140–5

55. Ferrero A, Maggi E, Giancotti A, *et al.* Regression formula for estimation of fetal weight with use of abdominal circumference and femur length: a prospective study. *J Ultrasound Med* 1994; 13:823–33

56. Kramer MS, McLean FH, Olivier M, Willis DM, Usher RH. Body proportionality and head to length 'sparing' in the growth-retarded neonates: a critical reappraisal. *Pediatrics* 1989;84:717–23

57. Kramer MS, Olivier M, McLean FH, Willis DM, Usher RH. Impact of intrauterine growth retardation and body proportionality on fetal neonatal outcome. *Pediatrics* 1990;86:707–13

58. David C, Gabriell S, Pilu G, Bovicelli L. The head-to-abdomen circumference ratio: a reappraisal. *Ultrasound Obstet Gynecol* 1995;5:256–9

59. Kurjak A, Breyer B. Estimation of fetal weight by ultrasonic abdominometry. *Am J Obstet Gynecol* 1977;125:962–5

60. Sumners JE, Findley GM, Ferguson KA. Evaluation methods for intrauterine growth using neonatal fat stores instead of birth weight as outcome measures: fetal and neonatal measurements correlated with neonatal skinfold thicknesses. *J Clin Ultrasound* 1990;18:9–14

61. Balouet P. Estimation du poids foetal. *Med Foetal Echogr Gynecol* 1994;17:10–17

62. Leroy B, Ngo C. Evaluation échographique du diamètre des membres foetaux. *Soirées Échogr Gynécol-Obstet* 1979;15:4–8

63. Warda A, Deter RL, Duncan G, Hadlock FP. Evaluation of fetal thigh circumference measurements: a comparative ultrasound and anatomical study. *J Clin Ultrasound* 1986;14:99–103

64. Balouet P, Speckel D, Herlicoviez M. Estimation échographique du poids foetal: intérêt de la mesure de la graisse des membres. *J Gynecol Obstet Biol Reprod* 1992;21:795–802

65. Naeye RL, Blanc W. Pathogenesis of congenital rubella. *J Am Med Assoc* 1965;194:1277–83

66. Barr M. Growth profiles of human autosomal trisomies at midgestation. *Teratology* 1994;50:395–8

67. Jacquemard F, Capella-Paulovsky M, MacAleese J, Mirlesse V, Daffos F. Apport de l'échographie du diagnostic et à l'établissement du pronostic des principales infections foetales. *Med Foetal Echogr Gynecol* 1994;18:16–23

68. Stuart B, Drumm J, Fitzgerald DE, Duigan NM. Fetal blood velocity waveforms in normal pregnancy. *Br J Obstet Gynaecol* 1980;87:780–5

69. Giles WB, Trudinger BJ, Cook CM. Fetal umbilical artery velocity waveforms. *J Ultrasound Med* 1982;1(Suppl):98–107

70. Campbell S, Díaz Recasens J, Griffin DR, *et al.* New Doppler technique for assessing uteroplacental blood flow. *Lancet* 1983;1:675–7

71. De la Fuente P, Galindo A, Olaizola JI. El Doppler en Obstetricia. *Actual Obstet Ginecol* 1989;1:9–22

72. Benson CB, Doubilet PM. Doppler criteria for intrauterine growth retardation: predictive values. *J Ultrasound Med* 1988;7:655–60

73. Carrera JM, Mortera C, Alegre M, Pérez Ares C, Torrents M, Salvador MJ. Fluxometría Doppler en la preeclampsia. *Prog Obstet Ginecol* 1989;32: 7–22

74. Carrera JM, Alegre M, Pérez-Ares C, Mortera C, Torrents M. Evaluación de las resistencias vasculares umbilicoplacentarias mediante el

análisis espectral de la onda de velocidad de flujo. *Prog Obstet Ginecol* 1986;29:321–9

75. Carrera JM, Alegre M, Pérez-Ares C, Torrents M, Mortera C. Evaluación de las resistencias vasculares uteroplacentarias mediante análisis espectral de la onda de velocidad de flujo. *Prog Obstet Ginecol* 1986;29:397–404

76. Carrera JM, Alegre M, Mallafré J, Pérez-Ares C, Torrents M. Control del embarazo gemelar mediante el análisis espectral de la onda de velocidad del flujo umbilical. *Prog Obstet Ginecol* 1986;29:599–606

77. Carrera JM, Alegre M, Torrents M. La fluxometría Doppler transplacentaria en los estados hipertensivos del embarazo. In Stopelli I, ed. *Gestosi*. Rome: CIC, 1987:89–94

78. Carrera JM. Control de la gestación diabética con Doppler. In Cabero L, ed. *Clínica Ginecológica*. Barcelona: Salvat, 1989

79. Carrera JM, Sanfeliu F, Blum B. Fluxometría Doppler umbílico-placentaria en el CIR. *IX Reunión Nacional de Medicina Perinatal*, Alicante, November 1987

80. Griffin DR, Cohen-Overbeek T, Campbell S. Fetal and uteroplacental blood flow. *Clin Obstet Gynecol* 1983;10:565–602

81. Thaler I, Manor D, Itskovitz J, *et al.* Changes in uterine blood flow during human pregnancy. *Am J Obstet Gynecol* 1990;162:121–5

82. Pourcelot L. Applications cliniques de l'examen Doppler transcutané. In Peronneau P, ed. *Velocimetric Ultrasound Doppler*, Vol. 34. Paris: Inserm, 1974:213–40

83. Creasy RK, Barret CT, De Swiet M, Kahanpaa KV, Rudolph AM. Experimental growth retardation in the sheep. *Am J Obstet Gynecol* 1972;112:566–73

84. Gu W, Jones CT, Parer JT. Metabolic and cardiovascular effects on fetal sheep of sustained reduction of uterine blood flow. *J Physiol* 1985;368:109–21

85. Trudinger BJ, Giles WB, Cook CM. Uteroplacental blood flow velocity–time waveforms in normal and complicated pregnancies. *Br J Obstet Gynaecol* 1985;92:39–45

86. Trudinger BJ, Cook CM. Doppler umbilical and uterine flow waveforms in severe pregnancy hypertension. *Br J Obstet Gynaecol* 1985;97:142–9

87. Bulfamante GP, Ferrazi E, Barber A, Pollina E, Pardi G. Doppler velocimetry of the uterine artery and ischemic–hemorrhagic lesions of the placenta. In Kurjak A, Chevernak FA, eds. *The Fetus as a Patient*. Carnforth, UK: Parthenon Publishing, 1994:419–24

88. Rizzo G, Arduini D, Romanini C. Fetal hemodynamics in growth retardation. In Kurjak A, Chevernak FA, eds. *The Fetus as a Patient*. Carnforth, UK: Parthenon Publishing, 1994:299–309

89. Campbell S, Pearce JMF, Hackett G, Cohen-Overbeek T, Hernandez C. Quantitative assessment of uteroplacental blood flow: early screening test for high-risk pregnancies. *Obstet Gynecol* 1986;68:649–53

90. Arduini D, Rizzo G, Romanini C, Mancuso S. Uteroplacental blood flow velocity waveforms as predictors of pregnancy-induced hypertension. *Eur J Obstet Gynecol Reprod Biol* 1987;26:335–41

91. Bower S, Schuchter K, Campbell S. Doppler ultrasound screening as part of routine antenatal scanning: prediction of preeclampsia and intrauterine growth retardation. *Br J Obstet Gynaecol* 1993;100:989–94

92. Montenegro CAB, Meirelles J, Fonseca AL, *et al.* Cordocentèse et evaluation du bien être foetal dans une population à très haut risque. *Rev Fr Gynecol Obstet* 1992;87:467–77

93. Montenegro CAB. Perfil hemodinamico fetal-Diastole-Zero revisitada. *J Brasileiro Ginecol* 1992;102:375–80

94. Thaler I, Weiner Z, Itskovitz J. Systolic or diastolic notch in uterine artery blood flow velocity waveforms in hypertensive pregnant patients: relationship to outcome. *Obstet Gynecol* 1992;80:277–82

95. Wallenburg HCS, Rotmans N. Prevention of recurrent idiopathic fetal growth retardation by low-dose aspirin and dipyridamole. *Am J Obstet Gynecol* 1987;157:1230–5

96. Trudinger BJ, Cook CM, Thompson R, Giles WB, Connelly A. Low dose aspirin therapy improves fetal weight in umbilical–placental insufficiency. *Lancet* 1988;2:214–15

97. Uzan S, Beaufils M, Bréart G, Bazin B, Capitant C, Paris J. Prevention of fetal growth retardation with low-dose aspirin: findings of the EPREDA trial. *Lancet* 1991;337:1427–31

98. Carrera JM, Mallafré J, Otero F, Rubio R, Carrera M. Síndrome de Mala Adaptación Circulatoria materna: Bases etiopatogénicas y terapéuticas. In Carrera JM, ed. *Doppler en Obstetricia*. Barcelona: Masson-Salvat, 1992:335–59

99. Di Renzo GC, Caserta G, Iammarino G, *et al.* The NO test in the management of hypertensive pregnancies and IUGR. *Ultrasound Obstet Gynecol* 1995;6(Suppl 2):29–35

100. North RA, Ferrier C, Long D, Townend K, Kincaid-Smith P. Uterine artery Doppler flow velocity waveforms in the second trimester for the prediction of preeclampsia and fetal growth retardation. *Obstet Gynecol* 1994;83:378–86

101. Jacobson SL, Imhof R, Manning N, Mannion V, Little D, Rey E, Redman C. The value of Doppler assessment of the uteroplacental circulation in predicting pre-eclampsia or intrauterine growth retardation. *Am J Obstet Gynecol* 1990;162:110–14

102. Bruinse HW, Sijmons EA, Reuwer PJHM.

Clinical value of screening for fetal growth retardation by Doppler ultrasound. *J Ultrasound Med* 1989;8:207–9

103. Chambers SE, Hoskins RP, Haddad NG, Johnstone FD, McDicken WN, Muir BB. A comparison of fetal abdominal circumference measurements and Doppler ultrasound in the prediction of small-for-dates and fetal compromise. *Br J Obstet Gynaecol* 1989;96:803–8

104. Fay RA, Ellwood D. Doppler investigation of uteroplacental blood flow resistance in the second trimester: a screening study for pre-eclampsia and intrauterine growth retardation. *Br J Obstet Gynaecol* 1992;99:527–8

105. Carrera JM. Intrauterine growth retardation. *VIII World Congress of Gynecology and Obstetrics (FIGO)*, Mexico, October 1976

106. Morrow RJ, Adamson SL, Bull SB, Ritchie JWK. The effect of placental embolization on the umbilical artery waveforms in sheep. *Am J Obstet Gynecol* 1989;161:1055–60

107. Morrow RJ, Adamson SL, Bull SB, Ritchie JWK. Acute hypoxemia does not effect umbilical artery waveforms in sheep. *Obstet Gynecol* 1990;75:590–3

108. Morrow RJ, Adamson SL, Ritchie JWK, Pearce M. The pathophysiological basis of abnormal flow velocity waveforms. In Pearce JM, ed. *Doppler Ultrasound in Perinatal Medicine*. Oxford: Oxford University Press, 1992

109. De Haan J. Fisiopatología de los cambios en los índices de flujo Doppler en la circulación fetal. In Carrera JM, ed. *Doppler en Obstetricia*. Barcelona: Masson-Salvat, 1992

110. Morrow RJ, Adamson SL, Bull SB, Ritchie JWK. Hypoxia, acidaemia, hyperviscosity and maternal hypertension do not affect the umbilical artery velocity waveforms in fetal sheep. *Am J Obstet Gynecol* 1990;163:1313–20

111. Laurini R, Laurin J, Marsal K. Placental histology and fetal blood flow in intrauterine growth retardation. *Acta Obstet Gynecol Scand* 1994;73: 529–34

112. Giles BG, Trudinger BJ, Baird PHJ. Fetal umbilical artery flow velocity waveforms and placental resistance: pathological correlation. *Br J Obstet Gynaecol* 1985;92:31–8

113. McCowan LW, Mullen BM, Ritchie JWK. Umbilical artery flow velocity waveforms and the placental vascular bed. *Am J Obstet Gynecol* 1987; 157:900–2

114. Rankin JHG, McLaughlin MK. The regulation of placental blood flow. *J Dev Physiol* 1979;1:3–30

115. Jackson MR, Walsh AJ, Morrow RJ, Mullen JB, Lye SJ, Ritchie JW. Reduced placental villous tree elaboration in small-for-gestational-age pregnancies: relationship with umbilical artery Doppler waveform. *Am J Obstet Gynecol* 1995;172: 518–25

116. Laurin J, Lingman G, Marsal K, Persson P. Fetal blood flow in pregnancy complicated by intrauterine growth retardation. *Obstet Gynecol* 1987;69:895–902

117. Carrera JM, Salvador MJ, Alegre M, Torrents M, Carreras E. El Doppler en Medicina Perinatal. Book of Abstracts of the *XII Reunión Nacional de Medicina Perinatal*, Valencia, 1990:465–515

118. Rotmensch S, Liberati M, Luo JS, *et al*. Color Doppler flow patterns and flow velocity waveforms of the intraplacental fetal circulation in growth-retarded fetuses. *Am J Obstet Gynecol* 1994;171:1257–64

119. Rochelson B, Schulman H, Fleischer A, *et al*. The clinical significance of Doppler umbilical artery velocimetry in the small for gestational age fetus. *Am J Obstet Gynecol* 1987;156:1223–6

120. Trudinger BJ, Giles WB, Cook CM, Bombardieri J, Collins L. Fetal umbilical artery flow velocity waveforms and placental resistance: clinical significance. *Br J Obstet Gynaecol* 1985;92:23–30

121. Brar HS, Platt LD. Reverse and diastolic flow velocity on umbilical artery velocimetry in high risk pregnancies. An ominous finding with adverse pregnancy outcome. *Am J Obstet Gynecol* 1988;159:559–61

122. Divon MY. Randomized controlled trials of umbilical artery-Doppler velocimetry: how many are too many? [Editorial]. *Ultrasound Obstet Gynecol* 1995;6:377–9

123. Jouppila P, Kirkinen P. Increased vascular resistance in the descending aorta of the human fetus in hypoxia. *Br J Obstet Gynaecol* 1984;91: 853–6

124. Illyes M, Gati I. Reverse flow in the human fetal descending aorta as a sign of severe fetal asphyxia preceding intrauterine death. *J Clin Ultrasound* 1988;16:403–7

125. Wenstrom KD, Weiner CP, Williamson RA. Diverse maternal and fetal pathology associated with absent diastolic flow in the umbilical artery of high-risk fetuses. *Obstet Gynecol* 1991;77:374–8

126. Valcamonico A, Danti L, Frusca T, *et al*. Absent end-diastolic velocity in umbilical artery: risk of neonatal morbidity and brain damage. *Am J Obstet Gynecol* 1994;170:796–801

127. Boehm F, Lomardi SJ. Reverse end diastolic flow velocity: reassuring biophysical profile and acute fetal demise. *J Matern Fetal Med* 1994;3:91–3

128. Torres PJ, Gratacos E, Alonso PL. Umbilical artery Doppler ultrasound predicts low birth weight and fetal death in hypertensive pregnancies. *Acta Obstet Gynecol Scand* 1995;74: 352–5

129. Hastie SJ, Danskin F, Neilson JP, Whittle MJ. Prediction of the small for gestational age twin fetus by Doppler umbilical artery waveform. Analysis. *Obstet Gynecol* 1989;74:730–3

130. Kurjak A, Rajhvain B. Ultrasonic measurements

of umbilical blood flow in normal and complicated pregnancies. *J Perinat Med* 1982;10: 3–16

131. Panella M, Santangelo G, Reggiani C, Gretter C, Mangano U. Flussimetria feto-placentare nell'ipertensione in gravidanza. In Stopelli I, ed. *Gestosi*. Rome: CIC, 1987:103–6

132. Reuwer PJHM, Sijmons FA, Bruinse HW. Intrauterine growth retardation: prediction of perinatal distress by Doppler ultrasound. Abstract Book of the *XI European Congress of Perinatal Medicine*. Rome: CIC, 1988:237

133. Gaziano E, Knox GE, Wager GP, Bendl RP, Boyce DJ, Olson J. The predictability of the small-for-gestational-age infant by real-time ultrasound derived measurements combined with pulsed Doppler umbilical artery velocimetry. *Am J Obstet Gynecol* 1988;158:1431–9

134. Kofinas AD, Penry M, Hatjs CHG. Compliance–weight. Deficit index. Combining umbilical artery resistance and growth deficit for predicting intrauterine growth retardation and poor perinatal outcome. *J Reprod Med* 1994;39:595–600

135. Zacutti A, Borruto F, Bottacci G, *et al.* Umbilical blood flow and placental pathology. *Clin Exp Obstet Gynecol* 1992;19:63–9

136. Griffin DR, Bilardo K, Diaz-Recasens J, Pearce JM, Wilson K, Campbell S. Doppler blood flow waveforms in the descending thoracic aorta of the human fetus. *Br J Obstet Gynaecol* 1984;91:997–1002

137. Arabin B, Saling E. Clinical value of multiple uteroplacental and fetal Doppler parameters. Abstract Book of the *XI European Congress of Perinatal Medicine*. Rome: CIC, 1988:253

138. Bilardo CM, Nicolaides KH. Cordocentesis in the assessment of the small-for-gestational age fetus. *Fetal Ther* 1988;3:24–30

139. Soothill PW, Nicolaides KH, Bilardo C, Campbell S. The relationship of fetal hypoxia in growth retardation to the mean velocity of blood in the fetal aorta. *Lancet* 1986;2:1118–20

140. Hackett GA, Campbell S, Gamsu H, Cohen T, Pierce JMF. Doppler studies in the growth retarded fetus and predictor of neonatal necrotising enterocolitis, haemorrhage and neonatal morbidity. *Br Med J* 1987;294:6–13

141. Marsal K, Nicolaides K, Kaminpetros P, Hackett G. The clinical value of waveforms from the descending aorta. In Pearce JM, ed. *Doppler Ultrasound in Perinatal Medicine*. Oxford: Oxford University Press, 1992:239–67

142. Marsal K, Persson P. Ultrasonic measurement of fetal blood velocity waveforms as a secondary diagnostic test for intrauterine growth retardation. *J Clin Ultrasound* 1988;16:239–44

143. Vyas S, Nicolaides KH, Campbell S. Renal artery blood flow velocity waveforms in normal and hypoxaemic fetuses. *Am J Obstet Gynecol* 1989;161: 168–75

144. Vyas S, Nicolaides KH, Bower S, Campbell S. Middle cerebral artery flow velocity waveforms in fetal hypoxemia. *Br J Obstet Gynaecol* 1990;97: 797–803

145. Arduini D, Rizzo G. Fetal renal artery velocity waveforms and amniotic fluid volume in growth-retarded and post-term fetuses. *Obstet Gynecol* 1991;77:370–4

146. Bilardo CM, Nicolaides KH, Campbell S. Doppler measurement of fetal and utero-placental circulation: relationship with umbilical venous blood gases measured at cordocentesis. *Am J Obstet Gynecol* 1990;162:115–21

147. Wladimiroff JM, Tonge HM, Stewart PA. Doppler ultrasound assessment of cerebral blood flow in the human fetus. *Br J Obstet Gynaecol* 1986;93:471–5

148. Van den Wijngaard JAGW, Wladimiroff JW, Reuss A, Stewart PA. Oligohydramnios and fetal cerebral blood flow. *Br J Obstet Gynaecol* 1988;95: 1309–11

149. Kirkinen P, Muller R, Huch R, Huch A. Blood flow velocity waveforms in human fetal intracranial arteries. *Obstet Gynecol* 1987;70:617–21

150. Rizzo G, Luciano R, Arduini D, *et al.* Prenatal cerebral Doppler ultrasonography and neonatal neurological outcome. *J Ultrasound Med* 1989;8: 237–40

151. Arduini D, Rizzo G, Romanini C, Mancuso S. Are blood flow velocity waveforms related to umbilical cord acid–base status in the human fetus? *Gynecol Obstet Invest* 1989;27:183–7

152. Soothill PW, Nicolaides KH, Campbell S. Prenatal asphyxia, hyperlactemia and erythroblastosis in growth retarded fetuses. *Br Med J* 1987;294:1051–3

153. Rizzo G, Arduini D, Romanini C, Mancuso S. Doppler echocardiographic assessment of atrioventricular velocity waveforms in normal and small for gestational age fetuses. *Br J Obstet Gynaecol* 1988;95:65–9

154. Reed KL, Anderson CF, Shenker L. Changes in intracardiac Doppler blood flow velocities in fetuses with absent umbilical artery diastolic flow. *Am J Obstet Gynecol* 1987;157:774–9

155. Groenenberg IAL, Wladimiroff JW, Hop WCJ. Fetal cardiac and peripheral arterial flow velocity waveforms in intrauterine growth retardation. *Circulation* 1989;80:1711–17

156. Rizzo G, Arduini D. Fetal cardiac function in intrauterine growth retardation. *Am J Obstet Gynecol* 1991;165:876–82

157. Ferrazzi E, Bellotti M, Marconi AM, Flisi L, Barbera A, Pardi G. Peak velocity of the outflow tract of the aorta: correlations with acid–base status and oxygenation of the growth-retarded fetus. *Obstet Gynecol* 1995;85:663–8

158. Rizzo G, Arduini D, Romanini C, Mancuso S. Doppler echocardiographic evaluation of time

to peak velocity in the aorta and pulmonary artery of small for gestational age fetuses. *Br J Obstet Gynaecol* 1990;97:603–7

159. Al-Ghazali W, Chita SK, Chapman MG, Allan LD. Evidence of redistribution of cardiac output in assymmetrical growth retardation. *Br J Obstet Gynaecol* 1989;96:697–704

160. Arduini D, Rizzo G, Romanini C. Fetal cardiac function in growth retardation. In Arduini D, Rizzo G, Romanini C, eds. *Fetal Cardiac Function.* Carnforth, UK: Parthenon Publishing, 1995:91–101

161. Fouron JC, Drblik SP. Fetal cardiovascular dynamics in intrauterine growth retardation. In Copel JA, Reed KL, eds. *Doppler Ultrasound in Obstetrics and Gynecology.* New York: Raven Press, 1994:281–90

162. Mari G, Deter RL. Middle cerebral artery flow velocity waveforms in normal and small-for-gestational-age fetuses. *Am J Obstet Gynecol* 1992; 166:1262–70

163. Block BSB, Llanos AJ, Creasy RK. Responses of the growth-retarded fetus to acute hypoxemia. *Am J Obstet Gynecol* 1984;148:878–85

164. Fouron JC, Teyssier G, Maroto E, Lessard M, Marquette G. Diastolic circulatory dynamics in the presence of elevated retrograde diastolic flow in the umbilical artery: a doppler echo-cardiographic study in lambs. *Am J Obstet Gynecol* 1991;164:195–203

165. Arbeille P, Patat F, Tranquart F. Exploration doppler des circulations artérielles ombilicale et cérébrale du foetus. *J Gynecol Obstet Biol Reprod* 1987;16:45–51

166. Fouron JC, Zarrelli M. Flow velocity profile through the fetal aortic isthmus. *J Matern Fetal Invest* 1992;2:122

167. Fouron JC, Teyssier G, Shalaby L, Lessard M, van Doesburg NH. Fetal central blood alterations in human fetuses with umbilical artery reverse diastolic flow. *Am J Perinatol* 1993;10:197–207

168. Teyssier G, Fouron JC, Bonnin P, Sonesson SE, Skoll A, Lessard M. Blood flow velocity profile in the fetal aortic isthmus: a sensitive indicator of changes in systemic peripheral resistance. Experimental studies. *J Matern Fetal Invest* 1993; 3:213–18

169. Bonnin P, Fouron JC, Teyssier G, Sonesson SE, Skoll A. Quantitative assessment of circulatory changes in the fetal aortic isthmus during progressive increase of resistance to placental blood flow. *Circulation* 1993;88:216–22

170. Goodwin JW. The impact of the umbilical circulation on the fetus. *Am J Obstet Gynecol* 1968; 100:461–71

171. Soifer SJ, Kaslow D, Ronm C, Heymann MA. Umbilical cord compression produces pulmonary hypertension in newborn lambs: a model to study the pathophysiology of persistent pulmonary hypertension in the newborn. *J Dev Physiol* 1987;9:239–52

172. Siassi B, Naves E, Stark C, Cabal LA. Normal and abnormal transitional circulation in the neonates with intrauterine growth retardation. *Pediatr Res* 1988;23:437A

173. Naeye RL. Cardiovascular abnormalities in infants malnourished before birth. *Biol Neonat* 1965;8:104–13

174. Rasanen J, Kirkinen P, Jouppila P. Right ventricular dysfunction in human fetal compromise. *Am J Obstet Gynecol* 1989;161:136–40

175. Mori A, Trudinger B, Mori R, Reed V, Takeda Y. The fetal central venous pressure waveform in normal pregnancy and in umbilical placental insufficiency. *Am J Obstet Gynecol* 1995;172:51–7

176. Appleton CP, Hatle LK, Popp RL. Relation of transmitral flow velocity patterns to left ventricular diastolic function: new insights from a combined hemodynamic and Doppler echocardiographic study. *J Am Coll Cardiol* 1988; 12:426–40

177. Reed KL, Appleton CP, Sahn DJ, Anderson CF. Human fetal tricuspid and mitral deceleration time: changes with normal pregnancy and intrauterine growth retardation. *Am J Obstet Gynecol* 1989;161:1532–3

178. Rizzo G, Arduini D, Romanini C. Inferior vena cava flow velocity waveforms in appropriate and small for gestational age fetuses. *Am J Obstet Gynecol* 1992;166:1271–80

179. Pinson CW, Morton MJ, Thornburg KL. Mild pressure loading alters right ventricular function in fetal sheep. *Circ Res* 1991;68:947–57

180. Bozynski MEA, Hanafy FH, Hernandez RJ. Association of increased cardiothoracic ratio and intrauterine growth retardation. *Am J Perinatol* 1991;8:28–30

181. Reed KL. The fetal venous system. In Copel A, Reed KL, eds. *Doppler Ultrasound in Obstetrics and Gynecology*, 1st edn. New York: Raven Press, 1995: 291–5

182. Hecher K. The fetal venous circulation. In Harrington K, Campbell S, eds. *A Colour Atlas of Doppler Ultrasonography in Obstetrics*, 1st edn. London: Edward Arnold, 1995:72–9

183. Kiserud T. The fetal ductus venosus. In Copel A, Reed KL, eds. *Doppler Ultrasound in Obstetrics and Gynecology*, 1st edn. New York: Raven Press, 1995:297–305

184. Jörgensen C, Andolf E. Four cases of absent ductus venosus: three in combination with severe hydrops fetalis. *Fetal Diagn Ther* 1994;9:395–7

185. Kiserud T, Eik-Nes SH, Blaas HG, Hellevik LF. Ultrasonographic velocimetry of the fetal ductus venosus. *Lancet* 1991;338:1412–14

186. Hecher K, Campbell S, Snijders R, Nicolaides

K. Reference ranges for fetal venous and atriventricular blood flow parameters. *Ultrasound Obstet Gynecol* 1994;4:381–90

187. Rizzo G, Pietropolli A, Bufalino LM, Soldano S, Arduini D, Romanini C. Ductus venosus systolic to atrial peak velocities ratio in appropriate and small for gestational age fetuses. *J Matern Fetal Invest* 1993;3:198

188. Kiserud T, Eik-Nes SH, Blaas HG, Hellevik LF, Simensen B. Ductus venosus blood velocity and the umbilical circulation in the seriously growth-retarded fetus. *Ultrasound Obstet Gynecol* 1994;4:109–14

189. Splunder IP, Huisman TWA, Stijnen T, Wladimiroff JW. Presence of pulsations and reproducibility of waveform recording in the umbilical and left portal vein in normal pregnancies. *Ultrasound Obstet Gynecol* 1994;4:49–53

190. Rizzo G, Arduini D, Romanini C. Pulsations in umbilical vein: a physiological finding in early pregnancy. *Am J Obstet Gynecol* 1992;167:675–7

191. Indik JH, Chen V, Reed KL. Association of umbilical venous with inferior vena cava flow velocities. *Obstet Gynecol* 1991;77:551–7

192. Nakai Y, Miyazaky Y, Matsuoka Y. Pulsatile umbilical venous flow and its clinical significance. *Br J Obstet Gynaecol* 1992;99:977–80

193. Vyas S, Campbell S. Doppler studies of the cerebral and renal circulations in small-for-gestational age fetuses. In Pearce JM, ed. *Doppler Ultrasound in Perinatal Medicine*. Oxford: Oxford University Press, 1992:268–78

194. Hudlicka O, Tyler KP. *Angiogenesis*. London: Academic Press, 1986

Fetal assessment

5

K. Maeda, J. M. Carrera and A. Muñoz

THE RISK OF HYPOXIA IN IUGR FETUSES

Small fetal size in cross-sectional examination, or intrauterine growth restriction (IUGR) in longitudinal fetal study, have been considered to show high risk for producing fetal hypoxia. Two categories of IUGR have been documented: fetal congenital anomalies and the restricted fetal growth caused mainly by fetal malnutrition due to placental abnormalities. Both of these *in utero* abnormalities can cause fetal hypoxia. It is easily understood that fetuses with congenital anomalies tend to develop hypoxia, because of several insufficiencies in the fetal organs, caused by an intrinsic factor in the fetus. Fetal hyponutrition is caused by an abnormality existing outside the fetus, i.e. maternal hyponutrition, placental insufficiency, etc. There is the risk of hypoxia in this category of IUGR caused by placental abnormality. Therefore, hypoxic risk should be taken into account in the management of all types of IUGR, particularly in the restricted fetal growth caused by placental insufficiency.

DEVELOPMENTAL MECHANISM OF HYPOXIA IN IUGR

Various congenital anomalies or chromosomal anomalies that involve IUGR tend to exhibit hypoxia, owing to the association of an anomalous circulatory system, particularly involving the heart, or an insufficient circulatory function. Another important cause is placental abnormality, in which fetal growth is restricted and fetal hypoxia is induced in an advanced stage of placental change. Its infarction, fibrin deposits and necrotic villi reduce the area for transfer of nutritive material and cause fetal malnutrition followed by fetal growth restriction. Placental

gas exchange will also decrease, owing to the reduction of the exchange area between the fetus and the mother, causing fetal hypoxia to appear in severe placental damage. However, the substance transfer function of placental villi should be further discussed, because usually the initial appearance is growth restriction, and the secondary change is the hypoxic finding, i.e. hypoxic fetal heart rate (FHR) changes frequently appear secondarily to growth restriction in fetuses with IUGR caused by placental abnormality.

According to the theories on blood flow in uterine vessels during pregnancy, there is trophoblastic invasion into the vessel walls of the spiral and radial arteries of the uterus in the first and second trimesters of normal pregnancy[1]. Uterine blood flow increases by the widening of the arterial cavities during pregnancy, but insufficient trophoblastic invasion of the arterial wall results in a narrow arterial cavity, causing slow arterial blood flow and reduced blood volume in the intervillous space. This change will produce various abnormalities, including placental infarction, fibrin deposits on the villous surface, fetal growth restriction and sometimes pregnancy-induced hypertension.

The other causes of fetal malnutrition are morphological and functional changes in the placental villi. Morphological changes include small villi seen in microscopic studies, and dystrophic and narrow villi observed by scanning electron microscopy in severely pre-eclamptic patients[2]. The reduction of end-diastolic flow and increased resistance and/or pulsatility indices detected by pulsed ultrasonic Doppler flow velocimetry of the umbilical artery in many studies on IUGR would be caused by the narrow fetal capillaries in the villi. In more severe flow pattern changes in the umbilical artery, absent or reversed end-diastolic flow (ARED) may be caused by the combination of the villus change and the induced circulatory impairment of advanced IUGR.

The function of substance transfer in the villi from maternal blood to the fetus differs according to the material passed through the villi; water is the easiest substance to pass the villi, and electrolytes are transferred by simple diffusion. Transfer of the gases oxygen and carbon dioxide is also by simple diffusion. Facilitated transfer is characteristic of glucose[3] and active transfer of amino acids[4]. The initial change of the villous function in the abnormal placenta is the decrease of facilitated diffusion of glucose and that of active transfer of amino acids, resulting in the restriction of fetal growth.

As the gases are transferred by simple diffusion, their transfer is maintained in the initial stage of fetal growth restriction, but the function decreases in more severe damage of the villi. In other words, fetal growth restriction precedes the reduction of gas exchange, and therefore restricted fetal growth usually appears before the hypoxia that develops in the final stage of placental damage. Mild placental abnormality produces no detectable hypoxia in spite of the presence of restricted fetal growth.

Some IUGR fetuses show FHR abnormality due to hypoxia only in labor, but fetal distress and possible fetal damage appear during pregnancy in the presence of the most severe placental damage. In the clinical course, IUGR is initially detected by ultrasound imaging, followed by a mild FHR change in a non-reactive non-stress test (NST). Signs of fetal distress together with blood flow abnormalities then appear, owing to increased hypoxia, which finally results in fetal damage. Amniotic fluid reduction appears, owing to reduced fetal urine production. Fetal breathing and gross fetal movements are suppressed. ARED flow of the fetal aorta and umbilical artery, associated with a non-reactive NST or fetal distress signs, develop (Table 1).

Table 1 Developmental mechanism of fetal hypoxia in placental abnormality

Reduced trophoblastic invasion of spiral and/or radial arteries, and no increase of end-diastolic flow in the flow velocity waveform of the uterine artery

↓

Reduced and slow blood flow in the intervillous space

↓

Placental infarction, fibrin deposits, necrotic villi, small dystrophic villi, decreased fetal blood flow in the villous capillaries, reduced end-diastolic blood flow and increased resistance and pulsatility indices of the umbilical artery

↓

Suppressed transfer of glucose, amino acids, fatty acids, etc., due to abnormal villous transfer function

Fetal malnutrition followed by restricted fetal growth

↓

Severe placental change, reduced gas transfer through the villi, reduction of oxygen supply to the fetus

↓

Non-reactive non-stress test, reduced amniotic fluid, reduced fetal breathing, reduced fetal movement, absent or reversed end-diastolic flow of umbilical arterial blood flow waveform

↓

Manifestation of fetal distress in fetal heart rate:
(1) under labor stress, in moderate hypoxia
(2) during pregnancy, in severe antepartum hypoxia

FETAL DISTRESS SIGNS IN FETAL HEART RATE DURING PREGNANCY AND LABOR

Severe fetal depression with impending damage of fetal organs and/or fetal death is caused by hypoxia, which needs interventional rapid delivery. It is detected by characteristic FHR changes[5–8], and the condition is usually called fetal distress. Although fetal distress is more acute and severe in the intrapartum than the antepartum stage, the following methods of FHR evaluation are applied either in the antepartum or in the intrapartum stage in the period after 28–29 weeks of pregnancy.

Continuous bradycardia

The shift of FHR into continuous decrease below 100 beats/min without recovery is the most serious state of fetal depression, followed by fetal damage, if it is caused by hypoxia. Fetal hypoxia is an important cause of bradycardia in various abnormalities, e.g. placental separation, umbilical vessel obstruction in the cord prolapse, fetal hemorrhage or maternal shock. FHR of 100–110 beats/min should be carefully monitored for further action.

Differential diagnosis Fetal cardiac abnormalities, e.g. complete atrioventricular block and sick sinus disease[9].

Continuous tachycardia

Fetal continuous tachycardia of 150–210 beats/min may be an early sign of fetal hypoxia and the later course should be carefully monitored. Other causes are the use of β-mimetics or atropine, maternal fever and fetal infection. Fetal tachycardia of 210–300 beats/min is usually a sign of fetal supraventricular tachyarrhythmia.

Severe variable deceleration

Deeply U-shaped transient FHR decreases are repeated. The onset and recovery are abrupt, and the shape and appearance are variable. The durations are more than 1 min, and the lowest FHR is less than 60 beats/min. The troughs of FHR decreases often show delay from the peaks of uterine contraction. The change appears more frequently in labor than in pregnancy. FHR variability is usually normal or excessive during and between the decelerations. However, severe decelerations accompanied by the loss of variability and rebound acceleration after the recovery (overshoot) is more ominous. The cause is fetal hypoxia due to the compression of umbilical vessels, e.g. prolapse of the cord, cord entanglement or compression of vasa

previa. Interventional delivery is appropriate in severe variable deceleration.

Differential diagnosis Mild variable deceleration, the duration of which is less than 1 min, the lowest FHR more than 60 beats/min. This does not need immediate delivery, because the cause is simple neural reflex due to mild umbilical cord compression. It needs careful monitoring, because it may change into severe deceleration.

Late deceleration

This is the repeated appearance of uniformly V-shaped transient FHR decreases with every uterine contraction, with a delay of more than 20 s with each contraction. The decelerations can be shallow in some cases. FHR variability is commonly lost during and between the transient FHR decreases. FHR acceleration does not appear on the FHR baseline in this case. Late deceleration appears less frequently than severe variable deceleration in labor, but its appearance is more common during the antepartum period. There is fetal hypoxia caused by placental abnormality, e.g. necrotic small placenta, severe placental infarction, or in pregnancy induced hypertension. Typical late deceleration needs intervention.

Differential diagnosis Early decelerations that are V-shaped decreases synchronized with each uterine contraction without delay, showing well-preserved normal variability. This is caused by fetal head compression, but not by fetal hypoxia. Mild variable deceleration sometimes resembles early or late deceleration, but the variable deceleration differs from the others by the instability of its appearance and onset, the U-shaped FHR decreases and no delay from uterine contractions. The variability is normal or large in mild variable decelerations.

Note Simple delay of transient V-shaped FHR decreases from uterine contractions with the preservation of normal variability in FHR baseline usually shows a favorable outcome, because the deceleration is caused by excessively active uterine contraction, or other acute mechanisms, but probably not by fetal hypoxia.

The loss of FHR variability

Small and fast FHR variations are not recorded between and during uterine contractions, irrespective of FHR deceleration. FHR acceleration also disappears. Typical late decelerations are associated with the loss of variability. It is ominous to observe both the loss of variability and overshoot in variable decelerations. This combination is usually caused by fetal hypoxia mostly during pregnancy, but also in labor. Very severe fetal brain damage (fetal brain death) was reported to have shown a totally flat, silent and straight FHR tracing.

Differential diagnosis Immature fetuses before 28–29 weeks of pregnancy. The resting fetus also shows decreased variability, but the normal fetus will show normal variability within 40 min after the onset of the active fetal state. The anencephalic fetus may show the loss of variability without hypoxia. The variability and acceleration are reduced or lost when the mother uses atropine, β-mimetics, sedative medication, or general anesthesia.

Sinusoidal FHR pattern

This pattern shows a regularly and slowly vibrating sine wave-like FHR baseline with a frequency of 2–3 cycles/min, and an amplitude of usually more than 10 beats/min. The vibrating FHR line is smooth, and loses the small and fast FHR variability that is noted in the normal fetus. The pattern appears in fetal hypoxia or severe fetal anemia, for example from Rh-isoimmunization, viral infection, thalassemia or hydrops.

Differential diagnosis Physiological appearance of a sine wave-like FHR change, which is associated with cyclic appearances of the clusters of fetal movements in the normal fetus, recorded by actocardiogram[10] (Figure 1), and/or observed by real-time sonography.

The pseudo-sinusoidal pattern is preceded and followed by a normal FHR pattern, and disappears in the active fetal state.

PREDICTION OF FETAL DISTRESS WITH ULTRASONIC DOPPLER ACTOCARDIOGRAM IN THE ANTEPARTUM STAGE

Ultrasonic Doppler actocardiogram

A moving object in the body produces a Doppler effect on the insonated ultrasound, e.g. fetal heart valves produce a Doppler signal with the frequency of about 400 to 1000 Hz when the ultrasound is 2–3 MHz; it is audible to the human ear from a loudspeaker, and the fetal heart rate can be recorded by processing of the fetal heart Doppler signal. The moving fetal body also produces an ultrasonic Doppler signal, although its frequency is as low as 40–60 Hz if the insonated ultrasound is 2 MHz. Maternal ambulatory motion and respiratory movement also produce ultrasonic Doppler signals with frequency lower than 10 Hz. Fetal movement is recorded after Doppler signals of the fetal heart and maternal motion are rejected by the band-pass frequency characteristics of the machine.

The actocardiogram utilizes a single ultrasonic transducer, which detects the fetal heart beat simultaneously with fetal movement. FHR is recorded by the high-frequency Doppler signals, and the lower-frequency Doppler signal is used for the recording of fetal movement, which is recorded by spike-like sharp and narrow signals (fetal actogram) on the lower channel of the cardiotocogram (CTG) (fetal actogram), instead of uterine contraction[11]. Simultaneous records of the FHR and actogram form the actocardiogram. There is automatic marking of fetal movements with the dot signals between the FHR curve and the actogram, and this is useful when the uterine contraction is recorded instead of the actogram.

The fetal active phase is clearly separated from the resting phase by the presence of many fetal movement signals on the actogram,

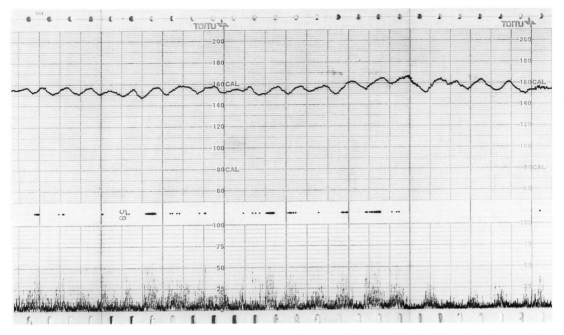

Figure 1 Pseudo-sinusoidal pattern recorded by actocardiogram. Sine wave-like baseline vibration noted on fetal heart rate (FHR) tracing (upper line) is synchronized with cyclic fetal movements on the actogram (lower line). The FHR before and after the pseudo-sinusoidal change showed a normal reactive pattern, and fetal outcome was normal

making the clusters (bursts) of fetal movement signals with irregular intervals (Figure 2). Many FHR accelerations appear simultaneously with the clusters of fetal movements, and the fetal movements precede, for a few seconds, the FHR accelerations[12]. In contrast, in the resting fetal state, no fetal movement signal or its cluster is recorded on the actogram, and no FHR acceleration is recorded. These findings are important in the differential diagnosis of a non-reactive FHR in the FHR NST. A physiological pseudo-sinusoidal FHR pattern is also differentiated from a pathological pattern by the cyclic appearance of fetal movement clusters synchronized with the sinusoidal changes of the FHR[10] (Figure 1).

Diagnosis of a truly non-reactive NST by fetal actocardiogram and the prediction of fetal distress

The objectives of the antepartum NST are to detect hypoxic fetal distress for the prevention of fetal death by the diagnosis of CTG signs (described elsewhere) and also to detect impending antepartum or intrapartum fetal distress that necessitates interventional delivery. Fetal distress is diagnosed by the detection of a non-reactive FHR that shows the disappearance of FHR acceleration during active fetal states characterized by fetal movements. However, the FHR baseline and the variability are normal, and no FHR deceleration is recorded in the non-reactive FHR.

IUGR fetuses tend to develop fetal distress because of remarkable hypoxia, which needs early delivery by Cesarean section during pregnancy and in early labor. Therefore, IUGR fetuses should be carefully monitored by CTG and other techniques. The actocardiogram is useful in the selection of high-risk cases that need intensive fetal monitoring because of impending fetal distress.

Therefore, the main purpose of the fetal actocardiogram is the detection of the non-

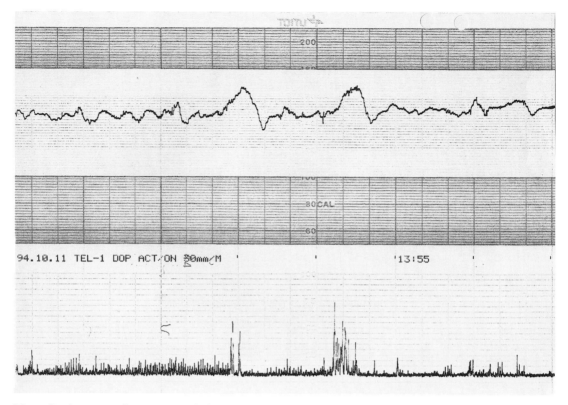

Figure 2 An actocardiogram recorded in the active fetal state. Fetal heart rate accelerations (upper line) are associated with fetal movement groups (lower line). Small and regular fetal movement signals are recorded in the left third of the actogram by sonographically confirmed fetal breathing movements

reactive FHR case, which should be repeatedly examined by CTG in short intervals or by continuous monitoring, possibly by other examinations including those of fetal growth, fetal breathing movement, amniotic fluid volume (by real-time sonography) and ultrasonic Doppler velocimetry to detect decreased, absent or reversed end-diastolic flow. Wireless telemetry using a combined transducer for fetal heart and uterine contractions is also useful for immediate detection of fetal depression, so that the pregnancy can be delivered with appropriate timing.

Inappropriate detection of a non-reactive FHR has been frequently reported with use of common CTG, because of many false-positive cases, mainly owing to the fact that FHR acceleration disappears in the resting fetal state where no fetal movement exists. Therefore, the diagnosis of a non-reactive

NST needs the CTG to be recorded during fetal movements. Although fetal movement is marked on the chart by the pregnant woman when she perceives the movement during the CTG examination, maternal perception is subjective; the time lag between the movement and the pressure of the switch greatly varies. The marking of fetal movement is therefore unreliable. Fetal movement is detected by the observation of real-time sonography, but still the mark of the movement depends on the observer. A more objective record of fetal movement without the time lag on the FHR is required for precise scientific evaluation. The fetal actocardiogram is useful for the purpose, because the FHR is evaluated when frequent fetal movements are recorded. A non-reactive NST is confirmed when there is no FHR acceleration recorded against the clusters of fetal movement signals, but it is not assessed when no fetal movement

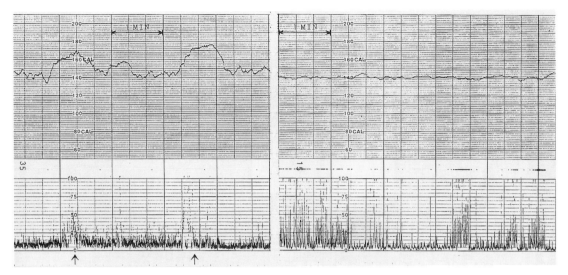

Figure 3 The left half of the figure shows the reactive actocardiogram recorded at 35 weeks of pregnancy, where fetal heart rate (FHR) accelerations are associated with fetal movement groups. The right half shows a non-reactive actocardiogram recorded at 36 weeks in an IUGR fetus. Frequent fetal movements appear in the actogram (lower line), automatic marking (middle) shows the presence of multiple fetal movements, but no acceleration is recorded in the the FHR (upper line). Severe variable decelerations appeared in this case 2 days after the actocardiogram, fetal distress was diagnosed, and a Cesarean section was carried out

signal is recorded on the actogram in the resting fetal state. It is recommended to wait for about 40 min before a subsequent NST, if no fetal movement is recorded but the pregnant woman reports normal fetal movements in usual life, because the longest duration of the normal resting fetal state is about 40 min[13]. The fetus can be stimulated by the vibroacoustic stimulator with the intention of being woken up if the examination time is limited.

We found a case of pregnancy-induced hypertension and IUGR that was non-reactive to the frequent movement signals in the actocardiogram. The baseline FHR was normal, variability was maintained and no deceleration was recorded, but the FHR acceleration was completely lost (Figure 3). We could not decide on the management, because the fetus showed the loss of acceleration, but other FHR parameters were normal. The patient was monitored with continuous CTG, and showed a fetal distress sign 2 days later. A diagnosis of fetal depression was made and Cesarean section was performed. Other IUGR cases showed

similar changes and a similar clinical course.

Teshima[14] collected 25 cases of pregnant women with a non-reactive NST recorded by actocardiogram, and 20 (80%) of these had IUGR. A fetal distress sign appeared in 19 cases (76.0%) of the 25 non-reactive patients in the further course of pregnancy and labor, 0–15 days after the detection of the non-reactive state on the actocardiogram, and 23 (92.0%) underwent Cesarean section. Most of them (13 cases, 68.4%) developed fetal distress within 5 days after the diagnosis. The 20 non-reactive IUGR cases were compared to 20 IUGR cases that showed a reactive NST. The non-reactive IUGR cases showed a shorter duration of pregnancy, lower birth weight, more fetal distress, more cases of low Apgar score, more Cesarean sections and more neonatal deaths, than the 20 IUGR cases with a reactive NST. The sensitivity for predicting fetal distress by a non-reactive NST diagnosed by actocardiogram was 81.0% and the specificity was 84.2% in the 20 truly non-reactive IUGR cases. The sensitivity increased to 93.8%, if the appearance of fetal distress was limited to the antepartum stage.

Therefore, the prediction of fetal distress was greatly improved by the use of the actocardiogram.

The combination of other methods of fetal well-being evaluation with the actocardiogram will be meaningful, because non-reactive NST cases detected by actocardiogram frequently showed ARED in the Doppler velocimetry of the umbilical artery and/or fetal aorta.

FETAL DISTRESS AND ULTRASONOGRAPHIC PARAMETERS

Cephalometric curve

It is obvious that the greater the deceleration in increases in biparietal diameter or head circumference measurements, the greater the likelihood of placental insufficiency. This is particularly evident in cases in which these parameters showed normal curves during the second trimester of pregnancy.

Fetal urine production rate

This is a parameter developed by Campbell and colleagues[15] which, based on fetal urine production, determines the amount of urine passed by the fetus during a specific period of time. In cases of IUGR, a decrease in perfusion in the territory of the aorta, and, in particular, in the renal vessels, reduces renal filtration and, as a result, fetal urine production. Wladimiroff and Campbell[16] have shown that in some cases of IUGR values fall below the confidence intervals expected for a specific week. We have obtained similar results in 56 cases of IUGR and 11 normal pregnancies (Figure 4).

In cases of IUGR type I and type III, usually without marked fetal hypoxia, the value of the fetal urine production rate fell below the lower limit of the confidence interval in only 33.33% and 30% of cases, respectively, while 70.58% of cases of IUGR type II, in which fetal hypoxia is common, did so.

Amniotic fluid volume

The importance of the quantitative determination of amniotic fluid volume in

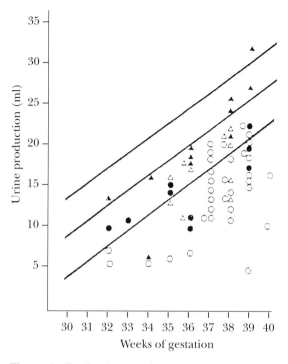

Figure 4 Fetal urine production rate in cases of intrauterine growth restriction (IUGR). Filled triangles, control group; filled circles, IUGR type I; open circles, IUGR type II; open triangles, IUGR type III

order to assess fetal condition has already been established. In cases of IUGR, a decrease in amniotic fluid volume indicates blood flow redistribution, which in turn leads to hypoperfusion of the kidney and decreased renal activity.

Fetal kinetics

Real-time ultrasound methods can help to determine the characteristics of fetal kinetics. When growth retardation is sufficiently marked to cause respiratory insufficiency, ultrasound imaging together with cardiotocographic monitoring usually detect decreases in fetal gross body movements and fetal breathing movements. These signs, however, appear long after abnormal cardiotocographic recordings have been detected[17–19]. Changes in the type of fetal body movement occur earlier. Apparently, before there is a quantitative decrease in fetal body

Table 2 Biophysical profile scoring: technique and interpretation (proposed by Manning and colleagues[25])

Biophysical variable	Normal (score = 2)	Abnormal (score = 0)
Fetal breathing movements	≥ 1 episode of ≥ 30 s in 20 min	absent or no episode of ≥ 30 s in 30 min
Gross body movements	≥ 3 body/limb movements in 30 min (episodes of active continuous movement considered)	< 2 episodes of body/limb movements in 30 min as single movement
Fetal tone	≥ 2 episodes of active extension with return to flexion of fetal limb(s) or trunk. Opening and closing of hand considered normal tone	either slow extension with return to partial flexion movement of limb in full extension or absent fetal movement
Reactive fetal heart rate	≥ 2 episodes of acceleration of ≥ 15 beats/min and of > 15 s associated with fetal movement in 20 min	< 2 episodes of acceleration of fetal heart rate or acceleration of < 15 beats/min in 20 min
Qualitative amniotic fluid volume	≥ 1 pocket of fluid measuring 2 cm in two perpendicular planes	either no pockets or largest pocket < 2 cm in two perpendicular planes

movements, an increase in so-called 'individual' movements is observed instead of more complex, stronger movements (rolling movements)[20].

Placental grading

Technical advances in the field of ultrasonography have permitted the observation of textural changes in the placenta *in vivo*. Sonolucent areas have been considered of particular interest in the assessment of fetal well-being in cases of IUGR[21,22]. Since 1980, placental images have been classified according to the classification of placental maturity changes developed by Grannum and co-workers[23]. The appearance of echo-spared or 'fallout' areas in the placental substance (grade III) are particularly relevant.

Ultrasonographic signs of a grade III placenta before week 35 were detected in 14.49% of cases of IUGR as compared to 6% in normal pregnancies. These differences were statistically significant in IUGR type II (17.64%; $p < 0.005$) and IUGR type III (14.28%; $p < 0.01$). As from week 35, the occurrence of echo-spared areas was twice as common in cases of IUGR (43% vs. 24% in

normal pregnancies), although this finding was statistically significant in only IUGR type II (58.82%; $p < 0.005$). Kazzi and associates[24] consider that the presence of a grade III placenta prior to week 35 should alert obstetricians to the possibility of IUGR. These authors reported a sensitivity of 62% and positive predictive value of 59%.

These images undoubtedly reflect pathological maturation changes.

FETAL BIOPHYSICAL PROFILE

One of the main reasons for using fetal biophysical profile schemes is the suspicion or evidence of IUGR. The combined use of different biophysical parameters both increases the sensitivity and the predictive value, and greatly reduces false-positive rates.

The biophysical profile proposed by Manning and colleagues

Manning and colleagues[25,26] developed a fetal biophysical profile based on a series of five basic variables: fetal breathing movements, gross body movements, fetal tone, fetal heart rate reactivity and amniotic fluid volume (Table 2).

Scoring

Each variable is assigned a score of 2, if considered normal, or 0, if considered abnormal.

The absence (abnormal) or presence (normal) of fetal breathing movements is assessed by ultrasound scanning of the fetal thorax and diaphragm along a longitudinal section of the fetus. Evidence of at least one episode of fetal breathing of 30-s duration, during a 30-min period of observation, scores 2 points. The absence of fetal breathing scores 0.

Gross body movements, defined as single or multiple, are assessed and counted by monitoring of the fetal thorax and upper and lower limbs. Detection of at least three movements of the body/limbs during a 30-min period of observation scores 2 points. The absence of body movements scores 0. Fetal eye movements, suckling, swallowing, etc. are also monitored but are not included in the profile; episodes of uninterrupted movement are assessed as one movement.

Fetal tone is assessed through ultrasound imaging of the trunk, limbs and hands of the fetus. Each episode of flexion/extension of the trunk or limbs scores 2 points, as does the opening and closing of the fetal hand. The absence of flexion/extension or opening and closing of the fetal hand scores 0.

Amniotic fluid volume is calculated by measuring the vertical diameter of the largest pocket detected. Although in the initial description, in 1980, Manning and associates[25] considered the largest pocket of fluid greater than 1 cm in two perpendicular planes to be normal (score 2), later however, in 1985, a vertical diameter of 2 cm was considered to be normal[26].

FHR reactivity is assessed by continuous cardiotocographic monitoring of the FHR during a period of 20 min. The observation of two or more FHR accelerations of at least 15 beats/min in amplitude and at least 30 s in duration associated with fetal movement(s) in a 20-min period scores 2 points; otherwise, 0 points are scored. If, during the first 20 min of monitoring, the trace is non-reactive, the examination will continue for another 20 min.

Manning and co-workers[27] believe that if the first four variables are normal, the biophysical profile test is complete. Only in those cases in which one or more variables are abnormal, is monitoring of FHR reactivity required.

Results

It has been shown that both the positive and the negative predictive values of the test are higher when variables are assessed in combination rather than individually[25,27–29] (Table 3). The false-negative rate is < 1% (between 0.5% and 0.8%) and, therefore, similar to the oxytocin challenge test. With its use, however, the number of false-positive results is considerably reduced.

Perinatal mortality is 10/1000 with scores of 10, rising to 600/1000 with 0 scores (27). In the experience of Baskett and colleagues[30] the rate of perinatal deaths was 0.3/1000 with scores 8 to 10 and 292/1000 with scores 0 to 4. The incidence of morbid perinatal outcome also increases when scores of the fetal biophysical profile are low (Table 4).

Although there are no statistically significant differences in sensitivity and specificity between the fetal biophysical profile and the NST, the positive predictive value of the biophysical profile is clearly higher. Moreover, the number of false-negative results registered is 4–6 times greater in the NST.

The progressive biophysical profile scoring method

New technological advances for use in antepartum fetal surveillance (vibroacoustic stimulation, Doppler velocimetry, etc.) which were not included in the fetal biophysical profile proposed by Manning and associates[25] in 1980, together with the aim to develop an integrated system of fetal monitoring applicable to all pregnancies, prompted us to design an alternative profile, the so-called

Table 3 Cumulative results of fetal biophysical profile for antepartum fetal assessment. (From reference 26, with permission)

Study population	Patients (n)	High risk (%)	Tests Number	Tests Normal (%)	Tests Equivocal (%)	Tests Abnormal (%)	Crude PNM n	Crude PNM Rate	Corrected PNM* n	Corrected PNM* Rate	False negatives n	False negatives Rate
Manitoba general population 1979–82	65 979	20	—	—	—	—	943	14.10	586	8.81	—	—
Manitoba prospective study	12 260	100	26 257	97.92	1.72	0.75	93	7.37	24	1.90	8	0.643
From reference 30	2400	100	5618	97.10	1.70	1.20	23	9.20	11	4.40	1	0.500
From reference 28	286	100	1112	94.00	3.50	2.40	4	14.00	2	7.00	2	7.400
From reference 32	150	100	342	94.90	2.00	3.10	5	33.00	4	26.60	0	0.000
Total	15 614	> 90	33 569	> 95	2.00	1.00	132	8.40	43	2.70	12	0.770

PNM, perinatal mortality; *corrected to exclude death due to lethal anomaly or Rh disease

Table 4 Last biophysical profile scoring result and normal perinatal outcome variable. (From reference 27, with permission)

	Last biophysical profile scoring result Normal	6	4	2	0	r^2 value	p*
Number of patients	6500	512	228	117	28		
Fetal distress (%)	12.8	24.3**	58.1	66.7	100**	0.9670	< 0.003
Admission to neonatal intensive care unit (%)	4	11.4**	28.8	40.2	83**	0.90	< 0.01
Intrauterine growth restriction (%)	3.4	4.4	28.8	41	75	0.92	< 0.01
5-min Apgar score < 7 (%)	3.7	11.4**	18**	30.8**	60.7**	0.89	< 0.02
pH recorded[†] (%)	4	14	27	26.5	53.6	0.98	< 0.001
Cord pH < 7.20[†] (%)	2.2	14.5**	26**	32.3	40**	0.98	< 0.002
Mean pH	7.36	7.34**	7.26**	7.22**	7.17**	0.97	< 0.01
Meconium (%)	8.7	20.3**	23.4	19.7	21.4	—	NS
Anomaly (%)	3.7	3.8**	4.1	4.3	14.3**	—	NS

*Calculated as linear regression of y or x as outcome variable; **significant increase compared with next highest score; [†]not a complete sample of all patients

'progressive biophysical profile'[31]. In the modified scheme proposed by our group, different testing procedures are carried out according to the characteristics of each pregnancy. The higher the risk, the more sophisticated the procedure used.

The progressive biophysical profile consists of three profiles (baseline, functional and hemodynamic), each of which varies in the degree of sophistication of the equipment used and the experience required of the examiner (Table 5). While the baseline biophysical profile is based on the results of conventional ultrasound imaging only, the functional biophysical profile requires the use of cardiotocographic monitoring and Doppler ultrasound equipment (continuous or pulsed) for the assessment of umbilical artery velocity waveforms. At the final step, the hemodynamic biophysical profile requires

Table 5 Progressive biophysical profile. (From reference 31)

	Baseline profile	Functional profile	Hemodynamic profile
Methods	ultrasound	ultrasound cardiotocography umbilical Doppler	ultrasound umbilical Doppler fetal Doppler
Parameters	fetal biometry	fetal movements	uteroplacental hemodynamic pattern

	amniotic fluid volume
	placenta grading
		tone
		cardiotocography patterns
		reflex activities (vibroacoustic
		  stimulation)
		umbilical Doppler (pulsatility
		  index)
			fetal hemodynamic pattern

the use of high-resolution ultrasound equipment including pulsed Doppler in order to assess velocity waveforms in fetal and uteroplacental blood vessels.

Altogether, the progressive biophysical profile includes all the biophysical variables that have been shown to be useful in screening for pregnancies that require special management and in predicting fetal condition, thereby enabling a prognosis and a management program to be established. Biophysical variables, however, are not determined simultaneously, as in the case of the fetal biophysical profiles proposed by Manning and colleagues[25] and Vintzileos and colleagues[32], but rather consecutively, depending upon the risk factors involved in each case. It is thus possible to institute a progressive, rational adaptation of the procedures available to the needs of each case. The greater the risk, the more complex the procedures used, the more time spent on examination, the greater the experience required of the examiner, and, inevitably, the higher the cost. The use of this strategy simplifies the patient's care and reduces the cost of medical attention without impairing the quality.

The baseline biophysical profile This includes the sonographic assessment of five variables; two provide fetal biometric data (cephalic area and abdominal area), another two provide data on the fetal environment (placental structure and amniotic fluid volume), and the fifth assesses the evoked fetal startle response or fetal movements in response to vibroacoustic stimulation (Table 6).

The functional biophysical profile Of the five variables included in this, two are assessed by cardiotocographic monitoring (cardiotocographic pattern evaluated by means of the Dexeus test, and evoked fetal startle reflex after vibroacoustic stimulation), two using real-time ultrasonographic imaging (fetal tone and gross body movements) and the last using Doppler continuous-wave ultrasound equipment capable of monitoring umbilical artery velocity waveforms (Table 7). Cardiotocography and ultrasound monitoring should take place over a period of at least 20 min.

The hemodynamic biophysical profile This includes the Doppler ultrasound assessment of velocity waveforms in the umbilical artery, descending aorta, common carotid artery and middle cerebral artery (Table 8). The hemodynamic biophysical profile should be carried out in pregnant women with previous abnormal functional profile scoring and pregnancy-induced hypertension. In cases of pregnancy-induced hypertension, early referral for fetal assessment by the hemodynamic biophysical profile is mandatory no matter what the result of the other two biophysical profiles.

Table 6 Baseline biophysical profile. (From reference 31)

	Score		
	0	*1*	*2*
Cephalic area	$< \bar{x} - 2$ SD	$< \bar{x} - 1$ SD and $> \bar{x} - 2$ SD	$> \bar{x} - 1$ SD and $< \bar{x} + 2$ SD
Abdominal area	$< \bar{x} - 2$ SD	$< \bar{x} - 1$ SD and $> \bar{x} - 2$ SD	$> \bar{x} - 1$ SD and $< \bar{x} + 2$ SD
Amniotic fluid index	< 5	5–8	> 8
Placental grading	IV	III	I–II
Acoustic stimulation*	non-reactive (< 7)	incomplete (7–8)	reactive (9–10)

*Scoring system, see Table 4: total score, 9–10, normal; 7–8, equivocal; < 7, abnormal

Table 7 Functional biophysical profile. (From reference 31)

	Score		
	0	*1*	*2*
Cardiographic pattern (Dexeus score)	< 7	7–8	9–10
Reflex activity (scoring system for vibroacoustic stimulation)	< 7	7–8	9–10
Fetal tone	absent	slow extension/flexion movements	rapid extension/ flexion movements
Gross body movements	absent	poor movements	rapid and numerous
Umbilical Doppler (pulsatility index)	absent end-diastolic velocity/reverse flow	> 95th centile	body movements < 95th centile

Total scores: 9–10, normal; 7–8, equivocal; < 7, abnormal

Table 8 Hemodynamic profile. Pulsatility indices. (From reference 31)

	Normal	*Abnormal*
Umbilical artery	< 95th centile	> 95th centile
Thoracic aorta	< 95th centile	> 95th centile
Common carotid artery	> 5th centile	< 5th centile
Middle cerebral artery	> 5th centile	< 5th centile

BIOCHEMICAL CORRELATION

The possibility of obtaining fetal blood by way of funiculocentesis[33] has allowed us direct access to the internal environment of the fetus in recent years, making possible the determination of various biochemical parameters (oxygenation, acid–base balance, etc.) that gives us information on the state of well-being of the fetus[34,35]. The few multicenter studies that are available[36] indicate that this method is a safe and easy procedure with a low rate of fetal mortality attributable to this technique.

Although the data in the literature are not unanimous, there appears to be a statistically significant association between the data obtained by Doppler velocimetry at the level of the umbilical, aortic, common carotid and median cerebral arteries[37–40] and the degree of hypoxemia and fetal acidemia.

Given that the data from velocimetry studies alone are not always accurate in determining the degree of fetal asphyxia, fluxometric studies that indicate a centralization effect should be followed by diagnostic funiculocentesis, according to various authors[41]. Pardi and co-workers[42] consider that fetuses with pulsatility indices exceeding the 95th centile should be investigated. In any case, the interpretation of the obtained results (pO_2, pCO_2, pH, etc.) should be carried out in accordance with gestational age, using existing standard curves.

We currently depend on evidence that there is a statistically significant correlation between fetal gases and velocimetric data arising from five vessels: the umbilical artery, aorta, common carotid artery, median cerebral artery and renal artery.

Umbilical artery

Velocimetric values that are altered in the umbilical artery seem to correlate with a notable percentage of low values of pO_2 and pH in blood from the umbilical vein in the majority of studies[40,43–47]. Nevertheless, as long as there are Doppler frequencies during diastole, the percentage of fetuses with hypoxemia, determined by funiculocentesis, is usually not greater than 25–30% of cases.

The situation changes drastically when the diastolic frequencies disappear (diastole 0). In this case 80% of the fetuses manifest hypoxemia, and 43% acidosis[45]. The figures recently reported by Montenegro and associates[43,44] are similar: 70.5% with hypoxemia, 66.5% with acidosis and 74% with asphyxia.

Thoracic aortic artery

Various studies have demonstrated that there is a positive relationship between velocimetric data in the descending thoracic artery and the degree of hypoxia, hypercapnea, acidosis and hyperlactacidemia in fetal blood obtained by funiculocentesis[37,48,49]. Nevertheless, because of the fact that there is a notable overlap between the data from the control group and the group of fetuses with IUGR, it is difficult to predict the fetal metabolic state with only the Doppler parameters.

Some authors[48,50] have even established a prognostic value of the pulsatility index and especially with zero diastolic flow in the flow velocity waveform of the aorta. Laurin and co-workers[48], using the aortic pulsatility index, predicted 63% of fetuses that would have fetal distress in labor, a figure that increased to 87% if, in addition, the flow velocity waveform was taken into account. Hackett and colleagues[50] demonstrated that the absence of diastole was accompanied by a significant increase in neonatal morbidity and mortality.

Common carotid artery

Bilardo and colleagues[39] correlated the observed differences between the pulsatility index values and the median velocity expected for the gestational age and those actually observed in the common carotid artery in 41 fetuses with IUGR with the biochemical data obtained by funiculocentesis (pO_2, pCO_2, pH, asphyxia index). The conclusion was that there was a significant correlation for the pulsatility index as well as for the median velocity and that the correlation coefficient was especially high with the hematological parameter being considered in the asphyxia index:

$$\text{Index of asphyxia} = -\Delta(pO_2 + 1.43 \, (\Delta pCO_2) - 180.2 \, (\Delta pH)$$

From velocimetric values obtained in the aorta (median velocity) and the common carotid artery (pulsatility index) another hemodynamic index was developed:

Index aorta–carotid = Δmedian velocity in aorta + 4.2 (Δpulsatility index in carotid)

In accordance with Vyas and Campbell[51], when the aorta–carotid velocimetric index is normal, the asphyxia index is normal. In contrast, when the velocimetric index is altered, 89% of fetuses have an asphyxia index situated at 1 SD below the mean, and 60% are situated below 2 SD.

Median cerebral artery

Vyas and co-workers[38] correlated the velocimetric results (median velocity and pulsatility index) obtained from the median cerebral artery in 81 fetuses with IUGR with data of the acid–base equilibrium in fetal blood, obtained from funiculocentesis performed 30 min after the Doppler study. The data were analyzed calculating the delta values of the velocimetric parameters such as the fetal gases. The conclusion was that there was a significant squared relationship between the delta-pulsatility index and Δpo_2, and also between the delta-pulsatility index and ΔpH.

In those cases in which the pulsatility index and median velocity were also determined, a statistically significant relationship was also confirmed between the delta-median velocity and Δpo_2 and ΔpH. In contrast, a consistent relationship between Δpco_2 and the delta-pulsatility index and delta-median velocity was not confirmed. On the other hand, these authors considered that the values arising from the median velocity in the median cerebral artery of small-for-gestational-age fetuses had a low rate of correlation with the value of the pulsatility index, attributing this fact to the existence of other factors that act on the flow: cardiac contractility, compliance of the vessels, blood viscosity, etc.

Renal artery

The same authors have studied a possible correlation between the velocimetric data of the renal artery and the biochemical parameters of blood from 48 fetuses that were normal with respect to chromosomes and morphology. The most notable conclusions from this study were: first, that no statistically significant relationship between delta-pulsatility index and Δpo_2 could be demonstrated in the whole group of fetuses, nor in those more than 24 weeks of gestation; and second, that there exists a significant relationship between these parameters in the group of fetuses of more than 24 weeks ($r = -0.368$, $p > 0.05$). These findings suggest that the vascular response to hypoxemia requires a maturation process before it is effective.

COMPUTERS IN THE ASSESSMENT OF FETAL WELL-BEING IN IUGR

Tools for the assessment of fetal well-being

There are three main tools in the assessment of fetal well-being. FHR is the most common subject in fetal monitoring. The first tool is the actocardiogram, which provides a simultaneous record of fetal movement signals and FHR, enabling study of the reaction of FHR to fetal motion; therefore, it is the best analytic tool of reactive and non-reactive NSTs. The second tool is ultrasonic imaging, which enables the monitoring of amniotic fluid volume, which is reduced in chronic fetal hypoxia. Gross fetal movement and fetal breathing are favorable markers of fetal well-being in real-time sonography. The third physiological tool is the analysis of the arterial end-diastolic waveform of pulsed Doppler flow velocimetry.

Computerized assessment of fetal well-being has been mainly carried out in the analyses of FHR and fetal movement, because electrical signals necessary for computer analysis are usually obtained from the output terminals of the FHR meter and the actographic amplifier.

Computerized assessment of fetal well-being

Dawes' computer system

The FHR signal is obtained by an ultrasonic autocorrelation monitor in this system[52]. The results of computer analysis are displayed on the computer screen, and a descriptive report is printed at the same time. Baseline heart rate, deceleration and other findings are demonstrated. Quantitative short-term variability is indicated by the difference in the beat-to-beat interval, considered to show a pathological state if the variability is reduced below the pre-set value. The main area of its application has been the fetus in the antepartum stage. The Oxford 8000® system is representative of Dawes' system.

Maeda's computer system

The ultrasonic autocorrelation fetal monitor is connected to a computer in this system[53,54]. Each FHR and contraction signal obtained every 5 min is automatically analyzed, and the computer reports the FHR baseline, number and amplitude of long-term variability, the number of accelerations in 5 and 20 min and the details of FHR decelerations, including the number in 5 min, the duration, the dip heart rate, the amplitude, the recovery time and the lag time in each deceleration. The number of uterine contractions and the area under the contraction curve in 5 min are also indicated. Uterine hyperactivity triggers an alarm if the area is larger than the pre-set value.

Second-step analysis and its report involve the recognition and warning of bradycardia, tachycardia, smooth baseline, loss of variability, a non-reactive state (loss of acceleration), late decelerations and other abnormal changes.

The third function is the report of the FHR score. The clinical bases of this were established in 1969 by the collection of abnormal FHR changes obtained with simple analysis in cases that developed neonatal depression. Every abnormality score was determined according to the frequency of neonatal depression, and abnormal scores were summarized in 5 min and then the FHR score was obtained. Fetal depression was suggested by 10 points or more on the FHR score[55]. The umbilical artery pH was significantly lower in patients with a high FHR score.

The fourth step analysis reports the fetal distress index. This increases and accumulates with a FHR score higher than 10, loss of variability, late deceleration and other severe FHR changes. The umbilical artery pH was considerably lower than 7.25 when the fetal distress index was 3 points or more within 30 min before delivery, while the umbilical artery pH was high when the fetal distress index was less than 3.

The affected state of the fetus is clearly demonstrated in these analyses and the system has been particularly useful in intrapartum fetal monitoring. Various warning signs are indicated on the panel or printout, including 'cord compression?', 'loss of variability', 'non-reactive?', 'transducer detachment?', 'fetal distress' and 'suspicious change'.

IUGR fetuses tend to develop fetal depression and exhibit fetal distress in an antepartum CTG. We analyzed normal CTGs in the NST by using an automated technique, and demonstrated normal ranges of FHR baseline variability and the acceleration during pregnancy (Figures 5 and 6). Lower values of variability and/or acceleration than the normal range in an antepartum NST indicated affected fetal well-being, and suggested the need of repeated fetal monitoring during pregnancy and intensive moritoring in labor. The Toitu MF-152® is a representative device in Maeda's system, and the program of automatic FHR analysis and diagnosis is incorporated in the up-to-date Toitu fetal monitor and central monitor.

Artificial neural network system

A neural network computer is composed of multiple units in the input, intermediate and output layers. The computer is trained by the FHR data obtained in the cases of typical outcome before it is used in decision making on the new subjects[56]. The system is objective because the computer is not programmed by experts' knowledge but educated on more than 500 occasions by the phenomena themselves.

The system was trained 1000 times by eight simple FHR parameters, including FHR baseline, variability amplitude, deceleration

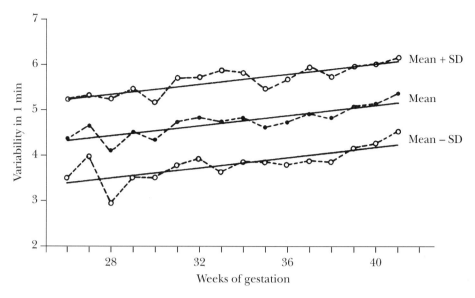

Figure 5 The frequency of long-term variability in fetal heart rate baseline in normal pregnancy. The values lower than the lower line (mean – SD) will be abnormal

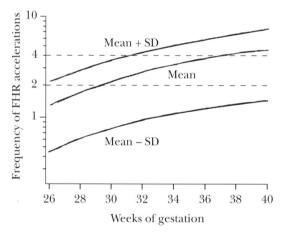

Figure 6 The frequency of fetal heart rate (FHR) accelerations (15 beats/min × 15 s or more) over 20 min (log scale)

number, duration, dip heart rate, recovery time, lag time of the deceleration and the presence of a sinusoidal pattern, obtained visually or automatically from the CTGs of normal, intermediate and abnormal cases in our studies.

The trained neural network computer analyzed newly obtained FHR data of 29 intrapartum cases that were classified into normal, suspicious and pathological groups according to the probability demonstrated in the final output of the neural network computer system. The results were compared to those obtained by our expert system in the same cases. The FHR score was low in the normal group, intermediate in the suspicious group and high in the pathological group, showing significant differences in each group. The fetal distress index showed a clear separation of the pathological group from the other groups.

In future, the CTG data of IUGR cases will be analyzed by the trained neural network computer, and an objective decision will be made from the analysis. A clinical system will be completed in the near future by the construction of parallel and hybrid systems of the neural network system accompanied by our expert system.

Other computer systems

There are various computer systems used in the analysis of FHR[57–60]. Di Renzo and associates[60] reported their chaos system in the difference of fractal data between normal and abnormal outcomes. Koyanagi and colleagues[59] demonstrated the changes in the probability distribution matrix composed of FHR baseline and the variability in *x* and *y* axes in 90 min or more in various stages of pregnancy. These analyses will be effective in the monitoring of IUGR fetuses in the future.

Cross-correlation of FHR and fetal movement signals

The FHR acceleration appears almost simultaneously with the cluster (burst) of fetal movement signals in the normally active actocardiogram. Therefore, the correlation of fetal movement and FHR acceleration is large in the normal case. The hypoxic IUGR case is, however, non-reactive and no acceleration appears against active fetal movement. Therefore, the correlation of FHR and fetal movement is small in the IUGR fetus that shows a non-reactive NST. However, there are various grades of the change in the abnormality. A more detailed and quantitative assessment of the hypoxic condition in IUGR fetuses was the objective of this study on the cross-correlation of FHR and fetal movement. Another purpose of this study was to confirm the precedence of fetal movement over FHR acceleration.

FHR and fetal movement signals were analyzed by the use of a personal computer.

The peaks of every movement signal were detected, and the data from three consecutive movement peaks were averaged. The correlation coefficient of FHR and fetal movement was calculated over 5 min, and, in addition, the movement data were delayed for −20 to +30 s, with the purpose of confirming the time relationship between FHR acceleration and fetal movements. The cross-correlation coefficient of the two signals obtained in 5 min was as high as 0.7 in the typical condition of the active fetal state, when the movement signal was delayed for 7 s. No correlation was observed in the resting fetal state, fetal breathing or fetal hiccups. The fetal sucking motion showed a moderate correlation[61].

These results suggested that fetal movement stimulated the fetus and caused a reactive FHR increase. Therefore, the cross-correlation coefficient of FHR and fetal movement was high, and the delay time of fetal movement was short in the normal fetus. The correlation coefficient may gradually diminish, and the delay time be prolonged, along the course of fetal deterioration due to hypoxia. Therefore, there is a possibility of quantifying the detailed progress of hypoxia in IUGR, and assessing the further usefulness of actocardiographic computer analysis in the monitoring of IUGR fetuses.

References

1. Bower SJ, Campbell S. Doppler velocimetry of the uterine artery as a screening test in pregnancy. In Chervenak FA, Isaacson GC, Campbell S, eds. *Ultrasound in Obstetrics and Gynecology*. London: Little Brown, 1993:579–86

2. Tsubaki O. Scanning electron microscopic observation on human placental villi of toxemias. *Acta Obstet Gynaecol Jpn* 1979;31:537–42

3. Widdas WF. Inability to account for placental glucose transfer in the sheep and consideration of the kinetics of a possible carrier transfer. *J Physiol* 1952;118:23–39

4. Iioka H, Moriyama I, Ichijo M. Amino-acids. In Takagi S, Sugawa T, Ichijo M, Mizuno M, eds.

Placenta – Basic and Clinical Studies. Tokyo: Nankodo, 1991:159–64

5. Hon EH. *An Atlas of Fetal Heart Rate Pattern*. New Haven: Harty Press, 1968

6. Maeda K. Physiology and physiopathology of the fetus. *Nippon Sanka Fujinka Gakkai Zasshi* 1969;21:877–86

7. Gibb D, Arulkumaran S. *Fetal Monitoring in Practice*. Oxford: Butterworth-Heinemann, 1992

8. Ingemarson I, Ingmarson E, Spencer JAD. *Fetal Heart Rate Monitoring: A Practical Guide*. Oxford: Oxford Medical Publication, 1993

9. Minagawa Y, Akaiwa A, Hidaka T, *et al.* Severe fetal supraventricular bradyarrhythmia without fetal hypoxia. *Obstet Gynecol* 1987;70:454–6

10. Ito T, Maeda K, Takahashi H, Nagata N, Nakajima K, Terakawa N. Differentiation between physiologic and pathologic sinusoidal FHR patterns by fetal actocardiogram. *J Perinat Med* 1994;22:39–41

11. Maeda K. Studies on new ultrasonic Doppler fetal actogram and continuous recording of fetal movement. *Acta Obstet Gynaecol Jpn* 1984;36:280–8

12. Takahashi H. Studies on cross-correlation coefficient between fetal heart rate and fetal movement signals detected by ultrasonic Doppler fetal actocardiogram. *Acta Obstet Gynaecol Jpn* 1990;42:443–9

13. Ohta M. Evaluation of fetal movements with ultrasonic Doppler fetal actograph. *Acta Obstet Gynaecol Jpn* 1985;37:73–82

14. Teshima N. Non-reactive pattern diagnosed by ultrasonic Doppler actocardiogram and outcome of the fetuses with non-reactive pattern. *Acta Obstet Gynaecol Jpn* 1993;45:423–30

15. Campbell S, Wladimiroff JW, Dewhurst CJ. The antenatal measurement of fetal urine production. *Br J Obstet Gynaecol* 1973;80:680–6

16. Wladimiroff JW, Campbell S. Fetal urine-production rates in normal and complicated pregnancies. *Lancet* 1974;1:151–4

17. Vintzileos AM, Campbell WA, Nochimson DJ, Wienbaum PJ. The use and misuse of the fetal biophysical profile. *Am J Obstet Gynecol* 1987;156:527–33

18. Vintzileos AM, Campbell WA, Feinstein SJ, et al. The fetal biophysical profile in pregnancies with grade III placentas. *Am J Perinatol* 1987;4:90–3

19. Ribbert LS, Snijders RJ, Nicolaides KH, Visser GH. Relationship of fetal biophysical profile and blood gas values at cordocentesis in severely growth-retarded fetuses. *Am J Obstet Gynecol* 1990;163:569–71

20. Sival DA, Visser GHA, Preechtl HFR. The effect of intrauterine growth retardation on the quality of general movements in the human fetus. *Early Hum Dev* 1992;28:119–32

21. Fisher C, Garret W, Kossoff G. Placental ageing monitored by scale echography. *Am J Obstet Gynecol* 1976;124:483–8

22. Catizone FA. Modelli ecografici di maturazione placentare. In Borruto F, ed. *Ultrasonografia ostetrica*. Verona: Libreria Cortina, 1981

23. Grannum PAT, Berkowitz RL, Hobbins JC. The ultrasonic changes in the maturing placenta and their relation to fetal pulmonic maturity. *Am J Obstet Gynecol* 1979;133:915–22

24. Kazzi GM, Gross TL, Sokil RJ, Kazzi NJ. Detection of intrauterine growth retardation – a new use for sonographic placental grading. *Am J Obstet Gynecol* 1983;145:733–7

25. Manning FA, Platt LD, Sipos L. Antepartum fetal evaluation: development of a fetal biophysical profile. *Am J Obstet Gynecol* 1980;136:787–95

26. Manning FA. Assessment of fetal condition and risk: analysis of single and combined biophysical variable monitoring. *Semin Perinatol* 1985;9:168–83

27. Manning FA, Harman CR, Menticoglou S, Morrison I. Assessment of fetal well-being with ultrasound. *Obstet Gynecol Clin North Am* 1991;18:891–905

28. Platt LD, Walla CA, Paul RH, et al. A prospective trial of the biophysical profile versus the non-stress test in the management of high-risk pregnancies. *Am J Obstet Gynecol* 1985;153:624–33

29. Manning FA, Baskett TF, Morrison I, et al. Fetal biophysical profile scoring: a prospective study in 1,184 high-risk patients. *Am J Obstet Gynecol* 1981;140:289–94

30. Baskett TF, Gray JH, Prewett SJ, Young LM, Allen AC. Antepartum fetal assessment using fetal biophysical profile score. *Am J Obstet Gynecol* 1984;148:630–3

31. Carrera JM, Mallafré J, Torrents M, Carrera E, Salvador MJ, Alegre M. Perfil biofísico progresivo. *Prog Obstet Ginecol* 1990;33:2

32. Vintzileos AM, Cambell WA, Ingardia CJ, et al. The fetal biophysical profile and its predictive value. *Obstet Gynecol* 1983;62:271–8

33. Daffos F, Capella-Paulousky M, Forestier F. A new procedure for fetal blood sampling *in utero*: preliminary results of 53 cases. *Am J Obstet Gynecol* 1983;146:985–7

34. Daffos F, Capella-Paulousky M, Forestier F. Fetal blood sampling during pregnancy with the use of a needle guided by ultrasound: a study of 606 consecutive cases. *Am J Obstet Gynecol* 1985;153:655–60

35. Nicolaides KH, Moya JMF, Snijders RJH. Cordocentesis en fetos pequeños para la edad de gestación. *Prog Diagn Prenatal* 1991;3:15–22

36. Hickok DE, Mills M, The Western Collaborative Perinatal Group. Percutaneous umbilical blood sampling: results from a multicenter collaborative registry. *Am J Obstet Gynecol* 1992;156:1614–18

37. Bilardo CM, Nicolaides KH. Cordocentesis in the assessment of the small-for-gestational age fetus. *Fetal Ther* 1988;3:24–30

38. Vyas S, Nicolaides KH, Bower S, Campbell S. Middle cerebral artery flow velocity waveforms in fetal hypoxemia. *Br J Obstet Gynaecol* 1990;97:797–803

39. Bilardo CM, Nicolaides KH, Campbell S. Doppler measurement of fetal and utero-placental circulation: relationship with umbilical venous blood gases measured at cordocentesis. *Am J Obstet Gynecol* 1990;162:115–21

40. Nicolaides KH, Bilardo CM, Soothill PW,

Campbell S. Absence of end-diastolic frequencies in umbilical artery: a sign of fetal hypoxia and acidosis. *Br Med J* 1988;297:1026–7

41. Campbell S, Soothill PW. Rule of fetal blood gas analysis in intrauterine growth retardation. *Lancet* 1990;336:1316–17

42. Pardi G, Ferrazzi E, Marconi AM, Lanfranchi A, Della Peruta S. Velocimetría Doppler de la arteria umbilical y de la arteria cerebral media y concentración de lactato en fetos con retraso de crecimiento. In Carrera JM, ed. *Doppler en Obstetricia*. Barcelona: Masson-Salvat, 1992:297–300

43. Montenegro CAB, Meirelles J, Fonseca AIA, *et al.* Cordocentèse et evaluation du bien être foetal dans une population à très haut risque. *Rev Franç Gynecol Obstet* 1992;87:467–77

44. Montenegro CAB. Perfil hemodinamico fetal-Diastole-Zero revisitada. *J Brasileiro Ginecol* 1992; 102:375–80

45. Nicolaides KH, Bilardo CM, Campbell S. Prediction of fetal anaemia by measurement of mean blood velocity in the fetal aorta. *Am J Obstet Gynecol* 1990;162:209–12

46. Arduini D, Rizzo G, Romanini C, Mancuso S. Are blood flow velocity waveforms related to umbilical cord acid–base status in the human fetus? *Gynecol Obstet Invest* 1989;27:183–7

47. Hsieh FJ, Chang FM, Ko TM, Chen HY, Chen YP. Umbilical artery flow velocity wavefoms in fetuses dying with congenital anomalies. *Br J Obstet Gynaecol* 1988;95:478–82

48. Laurin J, Lingman G, Marsal K, Persson P. Fetal blood flow in pregnancy complicated by intrauterine growth retardation. *Obstet Gynecol* 1987;69:895–902

49. Soothill PW, Nicolaides KH, Bilardo C, Campbell S. The relationship of fetal hypoxia in growth retardation to the mean velocity of blood in the fetal aorta. *Lancet* 1986;2:1118–20

50. Hackett GA, Campbell S, Gamsu H, Cohen T, Pierce JMF. Doppler studies in the growth retarded fetus and predictor of neonatal necrotising enterocolitis, haemorrhage and neonatal morbidity. *Br Med J* 1987;294:6–13

51. Vyas S, Campbell S. Doppler studies of the cerebral and renal circulations in small-for-gestational age fetuses. In Pearce JM, ed. *Doppler Ultrasound in Perinatal Medicine*. Oxford: Oxford University Press, 1992:268–78

52. Wickham PJD, Dawes GS, Belcher R. Development of methods for quantitative analysis of fetal heart rate. *J Biomed Eng* 1983;5:302–8

53. Maeda K, Arima T, Tatsumura M, Nagasawa T. Computer-aided fetal heart rate analysis and automatic fetal distress diagnosis during labor and pregnancy utilizing external technique in fetal monitoring. In Lindburg AB, Kaihara S, eds. *MEDINFO 80, Proceedings of the 3rd World Conference on Medical Informatics*. North Holland, 1980:1214

54. Maeda K. Computerized analysis of cardio-tocograms and fetal movements. B*aillière's Clin Obstet Gynaecol* 1990;4:797–813

55. Maeda K, Kimura S, *et al. Pathophysiology of Fetus*. Fukuoka: Fukuoka Printing, 1969

56. Maeda K, Noguchi Y. Neural network analysis of fetal heart rate. In Cosmi EV, ed. *The Place for New Technologies in Gynecology, Obstetrics and Perinatology. Proceedings of the International Symposium on Perinatal Medicine and Human Reproduction*. Bologna: Monduzzi Editore, 1995: 95–101

57. Arduini D, Rizzo G, Romanini C. Computerized analysis of fetal heart rate in normal and growth-retarded fetuses. In Kurjak A, Chervenak FA, eds. *The Fetus As a Patient, Advances in Diagnosis and Therapy*. Carnforth, UK: Parthenon Publishing, 1994:289–97

58. Van Alphen M, Waagenvoort AM, Van Geijn H. Quantitative intrapartum CTG analysis. In Cosmi EV, Di Renzo GC, eds. *Current Progress in Perinatal Medicine. Proceedings of the 2nd World Congress on Perinatal Medicine*. Carnforth, UK: Parthenon Publishing, 1993:805–11

59. Koyanagi T, Yoshizato T, Horimoto N, *et al.* Fetal heart rate variation described using a probability distribution matrix. *Int J Bio-Med Comput* 1994; 35:25–37

60. Di Renzo GC, Montani M, Fioriti V, Clerici G, Cosmi EV. Fractal analysis: a new method for evaluating fetal heart rate variability. *J Perinat Med* 1996;24:261–9

61. Takahashi H. Studies on cross-correlation coefficient between fetal heart rate and fetal movement signals detected by ultrasonic Doppler fetal actocardiogram. *Acta Obstet Gynaecol Jpn* 1993;45:423–36

Natural history of fetal compromise in intrauterine growth restriction

6

J. M. Carrera, C. Mortera and C. Comas

INTRODUCTION

The reduction in the number of functional arterioles in the tertiary villi gradually increases umbilical artery resistance with a subsequent decrease in po_2 in the umbilical vein. Both facts, at a specific moment in time, give rise to redistribution of blood flow, i.e. centralization of blood flow. The most highly oxygenated blood is distributed through vital organs (brain, heart, adrenal glands), while, as a result of vasoconstriction, blood flow to organs that are considered to be less vital is restricted (digestive system, lungs, skin, skeleton).

The redistribution or centralization of blood flow has been studied in experimental animals, in particular by Rudolph and Heymann[1] and Johnson and colleagues[2] in sheep, and by Berhman and associates[3] in fetal primates. In most cases, blood flow redistribution was assessed by injecting radioactively labelled microspheres, and hypoxemia and acidosis were induced by different procedures, such as maternal breathing of a mixture low in oxygen, hypotension, partial umbilical compression using clamps and microembolization of the umbilical arteries. In all cases the aforementioned pattern of redistribution of blood flow was confirmed. It is worth pointing out, however, that when fetal hypoxemia occurred as a result of maternal hypoxemia, not only did cardiac and cerebral blood perfusion increase but umbilical artery blood flow also increased significantly. This did not occur when fetal asphyxia was induced by microembolization of the umbilical arteries, a condition similar to that encountered in human fetuses with placental lesions[4,5].

ULTRASONIC STAGES

Four stages with relatively well-defined hemodynamic, biophysical and biochemical patterns can be distinguished by Doppler ultrasound studies in the compromised fetus with intrauterine growth restriction (IUGR).

Silent stage of increase in vascular resistance

Physiopathological basis The progressive impairment of the villous microcirculation is reflected in Doppler velocimetry of the umbilical artery (changes in the pulsatility index) only when more than 50% of villous arterioles are affected[6]. Until then, the theoretical deficit in gas exchange is maintained by the reserve capacity of the placenta as long as the maternal blood supply continue to be acceptable[7].

Doppler hemodynamic profile For a period of time, usually 3 to 6 weeks, fetal hemodynamic profiles are normal. Umbilical artery velocity waveforms show a positive blood flow pattern throughout the cardiac cycle and pulsatility, resistance or conductance values are within the confidence intervals. These are the umbilical artery velocity waveforms described by Laurin and associates[8,9] as type 0, with strictly passive diastolic flow. Doppler velocimetry of the remaining fetal blood vessels (descending aorta, common carotid artery, middle cerebral artery) also shows morphologically normal velocity waveforms with pulsatility indices within safety margins of each centile curve.

Doppler velocimetry in 82 cases of IUGR confirmed at birth showed that, in 36 cases

Table 1 Doppler velocimetry of umbilical artery pulsatility index (PI) and fetal hemodynamic profile (FHP) in 82 cases of intrauterine growth restriction confirmed at birth, with fetal mortality and pH of blood from the umbilical artery

	Cases		Fetal mortality		pH < 7.20	
	n	%	n	%	n	%
PI normal, FHP normal	36	43.9	0	0.0	6	16.6
PI normal, FHP abnormal	0	0.0	—	—	—	—
PI abnormal, FHP normal	22	26.8	0	0.0	8	36.4
PI abnormal, FHP abnormal	24	29.2	6	25.0	15	83.3
Total	82	100.0	6	7.3	29	38.2

(43.9%), the pulsatility index of the umbilical artery was normal. In none of these cases did the study of other fetal blood vessels show any abnormalities. For this reason, in-depth fetal hemodynamic study when umbilical waveforms are normal seems to be unnecessary (Table 1).

Biophysical correlation Both cardiotocographic recordings and other parameters included in the fetal biophysical profile are normal.

Biochemical correlation The study of fetal blood gases obtained at cordocentesis is normal. In our experience, this type of study is unwarranted when Doppler velocimetry gives normal results. Normal standardized curves have been developed using data obtained in cordocentesis protocols which have been indicated in circumstances other than those intervening in fetal distress (e.g. study of fetal karyotype, diagnosis of fetal infection).

Obstetric outcome There is no increase in the perinatal mortality rate and the percentage of IUGR is still not significantly high.

Decrease in umbilical blood flow

The decrease in umbilical blood flow is the first objective sign of chronic fetal compromise as a result of placental insufficiency.

Physiopathological basis As Trudinger[6] has shown in a mathematical model, the functional obstruction of over 50% of placental blood vessels causes umbilical artery velocity waveforms to be clearly abnormal (Figure 1).

Although it has been stated that the umbilical artery is not always the first vessel to be affected, in our experience and in that of other authors[10–13] the increase in umbilical artery resistance is usually the first apparent hemodynamic sign when there are placental lesions affecting the villous microcirculation. In only 15–20% of fetuses with IUGR of placental origin can the sudden decrease in po_2 cause an increase in the aortic and/or cerebral pulsatility index (mediated by aortic and carotid chemoreceptors) that precedes and/or is greater than that observed in the umbilical artery. On the other hand, it is also possible to detected abnormal pulsatility index values in the aorta or cerebral arteries prior to changes in umbilical blood flow, when the cause of fetal compromise is to be found in anomalies in the maternal environment (e.g. hypoxemia due to cardiopulmonary disease, severe nutrient deficiency, severe anemia) or in maternal circulatory hemodynamics (e.g. acute hypertensive episodes). In these cases, even umbilical conductance may increase.

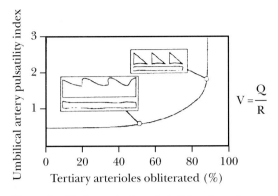

Figure 1 Mathematical model of Trudinger[6]

$$V = \frac{Q}{R}$$

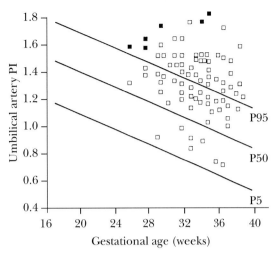

Figure 2 Umbilical artery: 56% of fetuses with IUGR (squares) present an abnormal pulsatility index (PI). Filled squares, IUGR and fetal death

Experimental studies have provided irrefutable evidence that a placental lesion is followed by decreased umbilical artery blood flow. In the studies of Morrow and colleagues[4,5] sheep fetuses were subjected to embolization of the villous microcirculation (plastic microemboli of 50 μm in diameter). Gradual changes in umbilical artery velocity waveforms similar to those detected in human fetuses with IUGR caused by placental insufficiency (decrease in diastolic blood flow, diastole 0, and, finally, reverse flow) were observed. The cause of the deterioration in umbilical artery velocity waveforms, therefore, must be found in the increase in the villous microvasculature resistance which, at the same time as it causes primarily umbilical artery flow to decrease, it also causes a gradual decrease in po_2 in the umbilical vein. Hypoxemia is, therefore, the result, not the cause, of umbilicoplacental hemodynamic changes. For this reason, a decrease in po_2 in the absence of placental insufficiency does not produce any changes in umbilical artery waveforms[4,5,14,15], nor are they affected by increased blood viscosity or an increase in maternal blood pressure[4,5].

Doppler hemodynamic profile For a certain period of time, the length of which largely depends on the rate at which placental lesions occur, a moderate increase in umbilical vascular resistance is the only sign of the onset of chronic fetal compromise. During this period, Doppler velocimetry of other fetal blood vessels (including the descending aorta) is usually normal. In our experience 56% of fetuses with IUGR present an abnormal pulsatility index of the umbilical artery, although in only 52% of these cases is an 'abnormal fetal hemodynamic pattern' found (Figure 2).

Doppler velocimetry of the umbilical artery shows positive flow velocities throughout the cardiac cycle, but the pulsatility index (or conductance) falls outside the acceptable range for the gestational age. A patent ductus venosus is the only hemodynamic compensatory mechanism – blood is directed from the liver to the heart – that can be observed by color Doppler. This shunting mechanism may delay centralization of blood flow for a period of a few weeks, but induces IUGR of the asymmetrical type[13].

Biophysical correlation All parameters of the fetal biophysical profile, including cardiotocographic recordings, are normal. Results of the vibroacoustic stimulation test and even the stress tests are also normal. These parameters are affected only when cerebral and/or fetal heart hypoxia occurs.

Biochemical correlation Oxygen supply to fetal tissues is normal. In our experience it is not necessary to carry out cordocentesis if the onset of centralization of blood flow is not confirmed.

Obstetric outcome According to our statistics for this group, there have been no cases of fetal death due to chronic fetal compromise, although there is a significant increase in the percentage of newborn infants that are small-for-dates. For this reason, 38% of newborns have pH levels < 7.20. In fact, there is a three-fold increase in the number of cases of intrapartum fetal distress, thus indicating a greater vulnerability of the fetus. Delivery is by Cesarean section in 30–40% of cases.

Centralization of blood flow

Physiopathological basis As umbilical artery resistance increases, there is a decrease in po_2 in the umbilical vein; when a certain level of po_2 is reached, in addition to dilatation of the ductus venosus, redistribution of fetal blood flow occurs so as to maintain oxygen supply to the fetal structures most sensitive to hypoxia. Redistribution of blood flow consists of the 'centralization' of blood flow as a result of selective vasodilatation of cerebral, cardiac or adrenal blood vessels and vasoconstriction of pulmonary, intestinal, cutaneous, renal or skeletal vessels. Doppler velocimetry reveals progressive increases in the pulsatility indices of the descending aorta and renal arteries, and decreases in the pulsatility indices of the common carotid and intracranial arteries.

These changes in arterial perfusion are mainly mediated by neuronal stimulation, either directly through stimulation of the vagal center or through chemoreceptors in the aorta and carotid arteries. Dawes and colleagues[16], in 1969, demonstrated that aortic chemoreceptors were sensitive to small reductions in oxygen levels in fetal lambs. It is likely, however, that vasoconstriction would be modulated by other factors, such as a direct effect of hypoxemia and acidemia on certain tissues through release of vasoactive compounds or catecholamines, or increase in the overall activity of the autonomic nervous system.

Although the chronology of these changes has not yet been established, it would appear that the first vessel affected after the umbilical artery and ductus venosus is the aorta. Increases in vascular resistance of the descending aorta are probably the result of the combined effect of several factors, such as an increase in vascular resistance of the umbilicoplacental vessels, reflex arterial vasoconstriction due to progressive hypoxemia and ultimately a decrease in myocardial contractility[17]. Lingman and colleagues[18] have suggested that there is an inverse relationship between myocardial contractility and the pulsatility indices of the umbilical and aortic arteries.

Hemodynamic Doppler profile Doppler velocimetry reveals an increase in the pulsatility index of the umbilical artery but also of the descending aorta and renal artery[19–23]. When vascular resistance reaches a certain level, a gradual decrease in diastolic velocity waveforms occurs in both vessels. A parallel decrease in pulsatility indices in the common carotid and cerebral arteries occurs, as a result of vasodilatation.

In our experience in 46 cases of IUGR with an abnormal pulsatility index of the umbilical artery, 52% of fetuses also showed abnormal increases in the pulsatility index of the descending aorta and 41.1% showed a decrease in vascular resistance of the middle cerebral artery (Figures 3–5).

Three stages in the process of centralization of fetal blood flow are frequently observed: the initial stage, the advanced stage and the terminal stage.

Initial stage The pulsatility index of the umbilical artery is elevated, but Doppler velocimetry frequency values continue to be positive throughout the cardiac cycle, even during the end-diastolic phase. On the other hand, common carotid artery velocimetry waveforms, for which diastolic frequencies are absent until week 32 to 34[24], recover diastolic velocity flow shortly after a moderate increase

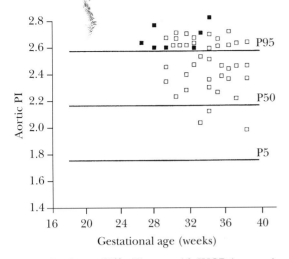

Figure 3 Aorta: 52% of fetuses with IUGR (squares) showed abnormal increases in the pulsatility index (PI). Filled squares, IUGR and fetal death

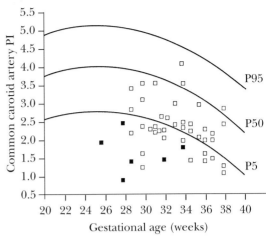

Figure 4 Common carotid artery pulsatility index (PI) in fetuses with IUGR (squares). Filled squares, IUGR and fetal death

in vascular intracranial perfusion occurs. This suggests that the decrease in the pulsatility index of the common carotid artery is largely due to a reduction in vascular resistance of the cerebral blood vessels.

During this initial stage, the assessment of the pulsatility index ratio of the umbilical artery and the middle cerebral artery (cerebral/umbilical Doppler ratio) could be particularly useful in providing evidence of the centralization of blood flow. Several authors believe that this is the best blood flow index to use in screening for IUGR[11,12,25].

Advanced stage Umbilical artery velocity waveforms show an absence of diastolic frequencies (the end-diastolic frequency disappears first, but subsequently the lack of blood flow is apparent in the whole diastole). According to Trudinger[6] this occurs when 80% of villous arterioles are occluded. Aortic velocity waveforms also exhibit absence of diastolic frequencies. At the same time, pulsatility indices of the common carotid artery and middle cerebral artery are at their lowest as a result of concurrent maximal vasodilatation of cerebral blood vessels (Color plate A).

Terminal stage In addition to arterial hemodynamic changes, signs of heart failure

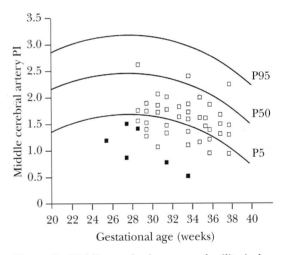

Figure 5 Middle cerebral artery pulsatility index (PI) in fetuses with IUGR (squares). Filled squares, IUGR and fetal death

become apparent in Doppler velocimetry of fetal venous blood flow, in particular elevated reverse blood flow in the ductus venosus and the vena cava (which coincides with atrial contraction) and venous pulsation in the umbilical vein (Color plate B).

An elevated reverse flow in the inferior vena cava indicates impairment of blood flow in the right atrium, which may be attributed to abnormalities in fetal heart rate or deficient atrial contractility[26–28]. Standardized normal curves of reverse flow in the inferior vena cava for each week of gestation[28] allow the differentiation of normal from pathological cases. Venous pulsation in the umbilical vein with apparent cyclical decreases in venous blood flow, coinciding with the absence of diastole in umbilical artery velocity waveforms, is also considered a sign of heart failure.

Venous signs of heart failure have the advantage over parameters that are exclusively assessed by ultrasonography, in that they are independent of the angle at which pulses of ultrasound are transmitted into the vessels, and do not require the calculation of the diameter or cross-sectional area of large blood vessels.

Biophysical correlation   In the initial stage of the centralization of blood flow, cardiotocographic recordings may still be apparently normal, and results of Manning's fetal biophysical profile considered to be normal or equivocal (scores 5 to 7). Changes in rest/activity cycles and a decrease in multiple fetal body movements ('rolling') are detected early[29]. Although there is an increase in abnormal results of non-stress tests in comparison with the previous stage, statistically significant differences between both stages have not been encountered.

In the advanced stage of the centralization of blood flow, there is a progressive impairment of fetal heart rate activity with the occurrence of late decelerations.

An abnormal pulsatility index of the umbilical artery usually precedes the occurrence of late decelerations in fetal heart rate by 9–60 days[30,31] (mean 2–3 weeks)[32–34]. Moreover, ultrasonography also shows a clear decrease in gross fetal movements, fetal breathing and fetal tone. The amniotic fluid volume can also decrease markedly (amniotic fluid index between 5 and 8)[35].

If all these parameters are evaluated according to Manning's fetal biophysical profile, a total score of < 7 is usually obtained. At this stage, the number of positive results obtained in oxytocin challenge tests is clearly significant, as are the results obtained in stress tests and vibroacoustic stimulation tests. Chronic fetal compromise, which, up to this point, was thought to be compensated, is now seen to be uncompensated.

Finally, in the late stage of the centralization of blood flow, cardiotocographic recordings not only reveal late decelerations in fetal heart rate but also a notable decrease in heart rate reactivity. These ominous recordings probably do not appear until 2–3 weeks after minimal values for the pulsatility index of the middle cerebral artery have been recorded. The time lapse depends on the ability of the fetus to compensate the reduction in its metabolic supply[33].

Total scores of the fetal biophysical profile are very low (always < 5), owing to abnormal results for each individual variable (marked decrease in fetal movements, fetal tone, etc.) and increasingly severe oligohydramnios (amniotic fluid index < 5).

Biochemical correlation   When abnormal Doppler arterial velocity waveforms are recorded not only in the umbilical artery but also in the remaining fetal arteries (descending aorta, common carotid, middle cerebral artery), low po_2 and pH levels are to be expected in fetal blood samples obtained at cordocentesis[11,12,29,36–38]. In fact, redistribution of blood flow begins only when fetal hypoxemia and acidosis occur. In the initial stage in which diastolic frequencies are still present in the aorta and umbilical arteries, there are usually no more than 25–30% of cases of hypoxemia. The situation changes dramatically in the advanced stage, coinciding with the disappearance of diastolic frequencies in Doppler velocimetry of the aorta and umbilical artery; in this case 80% of fetuses present clear signs of hypoxemia and 43% of acidosis[37].

Similar figures have been reported by Montenegro and co-workers[11,12]: fetal hypoxemia 70.3% of cases; fetal acidosis 66.6%; and fetal asphyxia 74%. In fact, most authors[39–41] consider that the absence of diastolic flow at this stage of redistribution of blood flow is evidence of an abnormal acid–base balance in fetal blood. In the late stage,

po_2 values in almost all fetuses are about -2 to -4 SD of the mean[42].

Obstetric and neonatal outcome A large number of fetal (250/1000) and neonatal deaths are found in this group, with a significant increase in the number of newborn infants with pH < 7.20 (83.3%). In our experience, the rate of Cesarean deliveries was 100%. The fetuses that survived showed a high incidence of complications (necrotizing colitis, hemorrhages, etc.) as a result of persistent vasoconstriction in specific organs[43].

Different authors[8,9,44] have reported that the absence of diastolic values in the aortic velocity waveforms predicts neonatal morbidity. Whilst the group of fetuses in which diastolic flow was absent suffered necrotizing enterocolitis (27% of cases) and hemorrhages in different organs (23% of cases) after delivery, these complications did not occur when diastolic frequencies were present[44].

Decentralization of blood flow

This is the term used by Montenegro and associates[11,12] to refer to the irreversible hemodynamic changes that take place after the centralization of fetal blood flow and which precede fetal death.

Physiopathological basis If hypoxia persists, a generalized phenomenon of vasomotor paralysis occurs. It may be postulated that the resulting condition may be similar to that described in experimental animals subjected to sustained and severe hypoxemia[45,46].

The cerebral blood flow is mechanically restricted, owing to the appearance of cerebral edema and the resulting increase in intracranial pressure. Cerebral edema is probably caused by local accumulation of lactic acid as a result of sustained anaerobic metabolism, which affects the permeability of the cell membrane, increases intracellular osmotic pressure and, finally, leads to edema and tissue necrosis.

In addition to hypoxia of cerebral centers, irreversible interference with control mechanisms of vascular tone in arterial vessels

also occurs (usually in extreme cases of hypoxemia at more than -4 SD of the mean)[42,47,48].

Doppler hemodynamic profile Mari and Wasserstrum[49], who reported the results of Doppler velocimetry in this condition, indicated that diagnosis was largely based on: first, confirmation of vascular resistance in the umbilical and peripheral circulation (aorta, renal artery) in the presence of reverse diastolic flow (Color plate C); and second, increases, after a brief period of stability, in pulsatility indices of intracranial arteries. These values may appear to be normal and cerebral artery velocity waveforms may be observed with no diastoles or with reverse flow.

The length of the time lapse between the onset of the process and intrauterine fetal death is not known, although it probably does not exceed 2–3 days and in many cases is a matter of only a few hours. This explains the difficulties found in detecting all these changes by Doppler velocimetry.

Biophysical correlation If, at this time, a cardiotocographic examination is carried out, a terminal pattern known as 'intrauterine fetal brain death' will be observed[50–55]. The recordings invariably show fixed fetal heart rate activity with no variability, and total absence of accelerations or decelerations, even when contractions are provoked by the oxytocin challenge test or vibroacoustic stimulation of the fetus. The fetal biophysical profile shows an immobile, atonic fetus and with very little amniotic fluid, although some cases with hydramnios have been reported[55,56]. The total score of the fetal biophysical profile is < 2. Cystic periventricular brain lesions (porencephalic cyst) or marked dilatation of the ventricles as a result of hypoxic necrosis are only occasionally observed by ultrasonography[55,57,58].

Biochemical correlation As has already been mentioned, if cordocentesis is carried out, extreme hypoxia is confirmed (po_2 values of less than -4 SD of the mean) and severe acidosis.

Obstetric outcome This is the phase that precedes death, so that fetal or neonatal death, when delivery is initiated, is the rule. Cesarean delivery is therefore considered to be unnecessary[55].

MANAGEMENT OF IUGR: TIMING OF DELIVERY

The decision as to the timing and the method of delivery should be taken with the following borne in mind:

(1) The objective data concerning fetal well-being (type of IUGR, absence or presence of congenital malformations, onset of centralization of blood flow, etc.);

(2) The degree of fetal lung maturity;

(3) The clinical features of each case (parity, underlying diseases, etc.).

In the case of IUGR type I (intrinsic or harmonious), with evidence, or likelihood, of fetal anomalies (trisomy or congenital malformations), whatever the results of tests to determine lung maturity or fetal hemodynamics, normal delivery may be contemplated. If the presence of congenital malformations has not been confirmed, the procedure to follow is that for extrinsic IUGR.

In the case of IUGR type II (extrinsic or disharmonious), different tests currently used in antepartum fetal surveillance should help to determine the most suitable time for delivery. Present knowledge and diagnostic possibilities afford two alternative approaches with regard to the timing of delivery.

The first is delivery when cardiotocographic recordings are abnormal and/or signs of chronic fetal distress are evident (decrease in fetal tone and fetal body movements, meconial staining of amniotic fluid, etc.). In this case, a high rate of asphyxia and perinatal morbidity and mortality may be expected[59,60].

The second is delivery at the onset of centralization of blood flow, in which case a high rate of prematurity of infants is expected. In order to minimize the latter risk, in particular if gestational age is less than 30 weeks, cordocentesis should be carried out to study fetal blood gases. This decision should be taken particularly when pulsatility indices in the aorta and umbilical artery are clearly abnormal, but diastolic frequencies are still recorded. If diastolic flow is absent or, more particularly, when reverse diastolic flow exists, fetal outcome is poor and cordocentesis is of little use.

In the case of mature fetuses or fetuses in transitional stages of maturity, delivery should always be instituted before disappearance of diastolic frequencies. Delivery when diastolic flow is absent may be too late, given the high percentage of acidosis (70%) and the high rate of perinatal mortality in this group.

References

1. Rudolph AM, Heymann MA. The circulation of the fetus *'in utero'*. Methods for studying distribution of blood flow, cardiac output and organ blood flow. *Circ Res* 1967;21:163–7
2. Johnson GN, Palahniuk RJ, Tweed WA, Jones MV, Wade JG. Regional cerebral blood flow changes during fetal asphyxia produced by slow partial umbilical cord compression. *Am J Obstet Gynecol* 1979;135:48–52
3. Behrman RE, Lees MH, Peterson EN, De Lannoy CW, Seeds AE. Distribution of the circulation in the normal and asphyxiated fetal primate. *Am J Obstet Gynecol* 1970;108:956–69
4. Morrow RJ, Adamson SL, Bull SB, Ritchie JWK. Ante hypoxemia does not effect umbilical artery waveforms in sheep. *Obstet Gynecol* 1990;75:590–3
5. Morrow RJ, Adamson SL, Bull SB, Ritchie JWK. Hypoxia acidaemia, hyperviscosity and maternal hypertension do not affect the umbilical artery velocity waveforms in fetal sheep. *Am J Obstet Gynecol* 1990;163:1313–20
6. Trudinger BJ. Doppler ultrasound study and fetal abnormality. In Drife JO, Donnan D, eds. *Antenatal Diagnosis of Fetal Abnormalities.* London: Springer-Verlag, 1991:113

7. Gruenwald P. The relation of deprivation to perinatal pathology and late sequels. In Gruenwald P, ed. *The Placenta*. Lancaster: Medical Technical Publishing, 1975

8. Laurin J, Marsal K, Persson PH, Lingman G. Ultrasound measurement of fetal blood in predicting fetal outcome. *Br J Obstet Gynaecol* 1987;94:940–8

9. Laurin J, Lingman G, Marsal K, Persson PH. Fetal blood flow in pregnancies complicated by intrauterine growth retardation. *Obstet Gynecol* 1987;69:895–902

10. Guidetti R, Luzi G, Simonazzi E, *et al.* Correlation between cerebral blood flow and umbilical blood flow in the fetus recorded with a pulsed Doppler system. Abstract Book of the *XI European Congress of Perinatal Medicine*. Rome: CIC, 1988:252

11. Montenegro CA. Perfil hemodinámico fetal-Diástole-Zero 'revisitada'. *J Brasileiro Ginecol* 1992; 102:375–80

12. Montenegro CA, Meirelles J, Fonseca AL, *et al.* Cordocentèse et evaluation du bien-être foetal dans une population à très haut risque. *Rev Franç Gynecol Obstet* 1992;87:467–77

13. Giorlandino G, Vizzone A. *Flussimetria ostetrica materna e fetale. Testo Atlante*. Rome: CIC Edizione Internationale, 1993

14. Morrow RJ, Adamson SL, Ritchie JWK, Pearce JM. The pathophysiological basis of abnormal flow velocity waveforms. In Pearce JM, ed. *Doppler Ultrasound in Perinatal Medicine*. Oxford: Oxford University Press, 1992

15. De Haan J. Fisiopatología de los cambios de los índices de flujo Doppler en la circulación fetal. In Carrera JM, ed. *Doppler en Obstetricia*. Barcelona: Masson-Salvat, 1992:89–97

16. Dawes GS, Duncan SL, Lewis BV, Merlet CL, Owen-Thomas TB, Reeves JT. Cyanide stimulation of the systemic arterial chemoreceptors in foetal lambs. *J Physiol* 1969; 201:117–28

17. De Vore GR. Examination of the fetal heart in the fetus with intrauterine growth retardation using M-mode echocardiography. *Semin Perinatol* 1988;12:66–79

18. Lingman G, Legarth J, Rahman F, Stangenberg M. Myocardial contractility in the anemic human fetus. *Ultrasound Obstet Gynecol* 1991;1:266–8

19. Marsal K, Lingman G, Giles W. Evaluation of the carotid, aortic and umbilical blood velocity waveforms in the human fetus. *XI Annual Conference of the Society for the Study of Fetal Physiology; Oxford*. Oxford: The Nuffield Institute, 1984:C33

20. Marsal K, Lindblad A, Lingman G, Eik-Nes SH. Blood flow in the fetal descending aorta: intrinsic factors affecting fetal blood flow i.e. fetal breathing movements and fetal cardiac arrhythmia. *Ultrasound Med Biol* 1984;10:339–48

21. Wladimiroff JW, Tonge HM, Stewart PA. Doppler ultrasound assessment of cerebral blood flow in the human fetus. *Br J Obstet Gynaecol* 1986;93: 471–5

22. Arabin B, Bergmann PL, Saling E. Simultaneous assessment of blood flow velocity waveforms in uteroplacental vessels, the umbilical artery, the fetal aorta and the common carotid artery. *Fetal Ther* 1987;2:17–26

23. Arabin B, Siebert M, Jimenez E, Saling E. Obstetrical characteristic of a loss of end-diastolic velocities in the fetal aorta and/or umbilical artery using Doppler ultrasound. *Gynecol Obstet Invest* 1987;25:173–80

24. Bilardo CM, Campbell S, Nicolaides KH. Mean blood velocity and flow impedance in the fetal descending thoracic aorta and common carotid artery in normal pregnancy. *Early Hum Dev* 1988; 18:213–17

25. Gramellini P, Folli MC, Raboni S, Vadora E, Merialdi A. Cerebral–umbilical Doppler ratio as a predictor of adverse perinatal outcome. *Obstet Gynecol* 1992;79:416–20

26. Indik JH, Chen V, Reed KL. Association of umbilical venous with inferior vena cava blood flow velocities. *Obstet Gynecol* 1991;77:551–7

27. Reed KL. Venous flow velocities in the fetus. In Jaffe R, Warson SL, eds. *Color Doppler Imaging in Obstetrics and Gynecology*. New York: McGraw-Hill, 1992:179

28. Rizzo G, Arduini D, Romanini C. Inferior vena cava flow velocity waveforms in appropriate and small-for-gestational-age fetuses. *Am J Obstet Gynecol* 1992;166:1271–80

29. Arduini D, Rizzo G, Romanini C, Mancuso S. Are blood flow velocity waveforms related to umbilical cord acid–base status in the human fetus? *Gynecol Obstet Invest* 1989;27:183–7

30. Reuwer PJ, Sijmons EA, Rietman GW, Van Tiel MN, Bruinse HW. Intrauterine growth retardation: prediction of perinatal distress by Doppler ultrasound. *Lancet* 1987;2:415–18

31. Bekedam DJ, Visser GH, Van Der Zee AG, Snijders RJ, Poelmann Weesjes G. Abnormal velocity waveforms of the umbilical artery in growth retarded fetuses: relationship to antepartum late heart rate decelerations and outcome. *Early Hum Dev* 1990;24:79–89

32. Arduini D, Rizzo G, Romanini C. Changes of pulsatility index from fetal vessels preceding the outset of late decelerations in growth retarded fetuses. *Obstet Gynecol* 1992;79:605–10

33. Arduini D, Rizzo G. Color Doppler studies of fetal circulation in intrauterine growth retardation. In Jaffe R, Warson SL, eds. *Color Doppler Imaging in Obstetrics and Gynaecology*. New York: McGraw-Hill, 1992:183

34. Griffin DR, Bilardo K, Diaz-Recasens J, Pearce JM, Wilson K, Campbell S. Doppler blood flow waveforms in the descending thoracic aorta of

the human fetus. *Br J Obstet Gynaecol* 1984;91: 997–1002

35. Phelan JP, Smith CV, Bronssard P, Small M. Amniotic fluid volume assessment with the four-quadrant technique at 36–42 weeks of gestation. *J Reprod Med* 1987;32:540–2

36. Nicolaides KH, Bilardo CM, Soothill PW, Campbell S. Absence of end-diastolic frequencies in the umbilical artery: a sign of fetal hypoxia and acidosis. *Br Med J* 1988;297:1026–7

37. Nicolaides KH, Bilardo CM, Campbell S. Prediction of fetal anaemia by measurement of mean blood velocity in the fetal aorta. *Am J Obstet Gynecol* 1990;162:209–12

38. Hsieh FJ, Chang FM, Ko TM, Chen HY, Chen YP. Umbilical artery flow velocity waveforms in fetuses dying with congenital anomalies. *Br J Obstet Gynaecol* 1988;95:478–82

39. Ferrazzi E, Pardi G, Bauscaglia M, *et al.* The correlation of biochemical monitoring versus umbilical flow velocity measurements of the human fetus. *Am J Obstet Gynecol* 1988;159: 1081–7

40. Tyrrell S, Obais AH, Lilford RJ. Umbilical artery Doppler velocimetry as a predictor of fetal hypoxia and acidosis at birth. *Obstet Gynecol* 1989; 74:332–7

41. Bilardo CM, Nicolaides KH, Campbell S. Doppler measurement of fetal and uteroplacental circulation: relationship with umbilical venous blood gases measured at cordocentesis. *Am J Obstet Gynecol* 1990;162:115–19

42. Vyas S, Nicolaides KH, Bower S, Campbell S. Middle cerebral artery flow velocity waveforms in fetal hypoxemia. *Br J Obstet Gynaecol* 1990;97: 797–803

43. Manning FA, Harman CR, Menticoglou S, Morrison J. Assessment of fetal well-being with ultrasound. *Obstet Gynecol Clin North Am* 1991;18: 891–905

44. Hackett GA, Campbell S, Gamsu H, Cohen-Overbeek T, Pearce JM. Doppler studies in the growth retarded fetus and prediction of neonatal necrotising enterocolitis haemorrhage and neonatal morbidity. *Br Med J* 1987;294:13–16

45. Myers RE, De Courtney-Myers GM, Wagner KR. Effects of hypoxia on fetal brain. In Beard RW, Nathanielsz PW, eds. *Fetal Physiology and Medicine.* London: Butterworth, 1984:419

46. Richardson BS, Rurak D, Patrick IE, Homan J, Carmichael I. Cerebral oxidative metabolism during sustained hypoxaemia in fetal sheep. *J Dev Physiol* 1989;2:37–43

47. Vyas S. Pulsed Doppler examination of the normal human fetus. In Pearce JM, ed. *Doppler Ultrasound in Perinatal Medicine.* Oxford: Oxford University Press, 1992

48. Vyas S, Campbell S. Doppler studies of the cerebral and renal circulations in small-for-gestational age fetuses. In Pearce JM, ed. *Doppler Ultrasound in Perinatal Medicine.* Oxford: Oxford University Press, 1992:268–78

49. Mari G, Wasserstrum N. Flow velocity waveforms of the fetal circulation preceding fetal death in a case of lupus anticoagulant. *Am J Obstet Gynecol* 1991;164:776–8

50. Adams RD, Prod'Hom LS, Rabinowicz TH. Intrauterine brain death. *Acta Neuropathol* 1977; 40:41–9

51. Gaziano EP, Freeman DW. Analysis of heart rate patterns preceding fetal death. *Obstet Gynecol* 1977;50:578–82

52. Van der Moer PE, Gerretsen G, Visser GHA. Fixed fetal heart rate pattern after intrauterine accidental decerebration. *Obstet Gynecol* 1985;65: 125–7

53. Nijhuis JG, Kruyt N, Van Vijck JAM. Fetal brain death. Two case reports. *Br J Obstet Gynaecol* 1988; 85:197–200

54. Nijhuis JG, Crevels AJ, Van Dongen PWJ. Fetal brain death: the definition of a fetal heart rate pattern and its clinical consequences. *Obstet Gynecol Surv* 1990;45:229–32

55. Zimmer EZ, Jakobi P, Goldstein I, Gutterman E. Cardiotocographic and sonographic findings in two cases of antenatally diagnosed intrauterine fetal brain death. *Prenat Diagn* 1992;12:271–6

56. Ellis WG, Goetzman BW, Lindenberg JA. Neuropathologic documentation of prenatal brain damage. *Am J Dis Child* 1988;142:858–66

57. Nwaesei CG, Pape KE, Martin DJ, Becker LE, Fitz CR. Periventricular infarction diagnosed by ultrasound: a postmortem correlation. *J Pediatr* 1984;105:106–10

58. Hill A. Assessment of the fetus: relevance to brain injury. *Clin Perinatol* 1989;16:413–14

59. Visser GH. Abnormal antepartum fetal heart rate patterns and subsequent handicap. *Baillière's Clin Obstet Gynaecol* 1988;2:117–24

60. Favre R, Nissand J, Messer G. Velocimetric sylvienne foetale. Critére d'extraction dans l'hypotrophic sévere. *J Gynecol Obstet Biol Reprod* 1991;20:699

Definition, etiology and clinical implications of macrosomia

J. M. Carrera and R. B. Elejalde

DEFINITION

Macrosomia is characterized by an acceleration of intrauterine fetal growth, resulting in infants with a birth weight in excess of 4500 g or above the 90th centile of population-specific growth curves.

ETIOLOGY

The etiology of macrosomia is believed to be multifactorial, although this condition is frequently observed in pregnancies complicated by diabetes mellitus.

Genetic factors

The main determinant of size in different species is genetic. Mechanisms that control growth, however, are poorly identified. It is considered that 20% of growth variation is attributable to fetal genotype, with maternal weight and height exerting a marked influence on the final weight of the fetus[1,2].

In only a small percentage of cases is macrosomia a part of certain genetically determined syndromes and, at the present time, no specific testing is available for the prenatal diagnosis of this subgroup of disorders.

In general, the literature concerning treatment of syndromes associated with macrosomia is quite confusing. Macrosomia-associated disorders are usually classified into three types. The first type includes those syndromes with generalized macrosomia (in which all parameters related to growth and physical development are affected) (Table 1). The second type includes those syndromes with macrosomia involving a part of the body. The third type includes those syndromes in which only one parameter (weight, height, skeletal development) is affected. We have classified the two last types

Table 1 Syndromes associated with generalized macrosomia

Present at birth	*Not present at birth*
Bannayan–Riley–Ruvalcava	familial rapid maturation
Beckwith–Wiedemann	familial high height
Elejalde	fragile X
Nesidioblastosis	gigantism/acromegaly
Perlman	congenital hyperthyroidism
Simpson–Golabi–Behmel	infantile hyperthyroidism
Sotos	Klinefelter
Overgrowth type Teebi	Marfan
Warkany (trisomy 8 mosaicism)	precocious puberty
Weaver	

into the subgroup of syndromes with partial macrosomia (Table 2).

The group of syndromes with generalized macrosomia present at birth exhibit some common features (weight and height are equally affected, mental retardation is usually present) and constitute the most homogeneous group of macrosomia-associated disorders because they probably share some pathogenetic mechanisms.

The reported prevalence rates of these syndromes are highly variable. The fragile X syndrome seems to be the most frequent with a prevalence rate between 1 in 500 and 1 in 1000 births. By contrast, Elejalde syndrome has only been described among members of a single family, so it can be assumed that its prevalence is lower than 1 in 100 000 births. Given the absence of population-based studies, it is difficult to establish the occurrence of these extremely rare disorders.

When signs of generalized or partial macrosomia are detected, it is very important to rule out the presence of these syndromes. In the majority of cases, early diagnosis will allow a number of therapeutic, and sometimes preventive, interventions of a series of complications directly related to the survival and quality of life of these patients. The following is a brief description of rare macrosomia-associated syndromes of clinical interest.

Beckwith–Wiedemann syndrome Since its first description, only 200 cases have been reported in the literature[3]. Infants with this syndrome show excessive birth weight (mean 4000 g), macroglossia, linear folds in the pinnae and omphalocele in a high percentage of cases. Hydramnios and prematurity are frequent. Macrosomia is mainly at the expense of muscular tissue and greater deposition of subcutaneous fat. Neonatal hypoglycemia is found in 30–50% of cases, and hyper-insulinemia is detected in most patients. Other common features include an increase in the number of erythrocytes, blood hyperviscosity and dyspnea, as well as mild to moderate mental retardation, which may improve if the condition is properly diagnosed

Table 2 Syndromes associated with partial macrosomia

Cutis marmorata telangiectatica congenita
Familial macrocephaly
Hemifacial microsomy/macrodactyly
Hemihyperplasia
Klippel–Trenaunay–Weber
Maffucci
Neurofibromatosis
Ollier
Patterson–David
Proteus
Seip–Berardinelli
Börjeson–Forssman–Lehmann
Cohen
Beals
Familial idiopathic obesity
Marshall–Smith
Subcutaneous lipomatous nevus
Prader–Willi
Macrosomia–microphthalmia–Teebi's cleft palate

and treated during the neonatal period. Neonatal complications are similar to those presented by infants born to diabetic mothers. An increase in the number and affinity of insulin receptors of erythrocytes has been reported and it has been suggested that the excessive growth results from an increased response to normal or slightly elevated serum insulin concentrations[3–5]. Neonatal hypoglycemia is often severe and may cause seizures. Treatment with hydrocortisone may reverse the clinical picture. The diagnosis should be suspected antenatally in a fetus with macrosomia, omphalocele and macroglossia[6]. Amniocentesis should be performed to identify the fetuses that are potentially carriers of aneuploidy.

Sotos syndrome This syndrome is characterized by macrocephaly, dolichocephaly and prognathism with moderate to severe mental retardation in 83% of cases. Sporadic cases of this disorder have been reported, although it may occur as an autosomal dominant disease. The glucose tolerance test is abnormal in 14% of neonates[7]. Prenatal ultrasonography reveals a fetus with excessive weight for gestational age and a higher head/abdominal circumference ratio (as found in asymmetrical or extrinsic intrauterine growth restriction).

Gillian Turner syndrome Gillian Turner syndrome is an autosomal recessive disease linked to the X chromosome, characterized by mental retardation, enlargement of genitalia and variable degrees of macrosomia. Cerebral gigantism may also be present.

Weaver syndrome This rare syndrome is characterized by accelerated skeletal development, unusual facies and campto-dactyly[8].

Nesidioblastosis This condition is characterized by diffuse proliferation of pancreatic islet cells with a relative increase of β cells. A disorder of islet organization preventing the usual paracrine regulation of insulin secretion by other hormones such as somatostatin has been postulated as the primary defect. The only effective long-term treatment is surgical excision of 95% of the hyperplastic pancreatic tissue. Although the etiology is unknown, it seems to represent an autosomal recessive defect of pancreatic development. Newborns are phenotypically similar to infants born to diabetic mothers, with macrosomia due to hypertrophy of muscular and subcutaneous tissue.

Fetal hormones

Fetal growth is controlled by the genome; fetal hormones translate genetic information into stimuli for growth, although the precise mechanisms controlling and regulating growth have not been clearly established.

Insulin This hormone plays an important role during postnatal life in carbohydrate metabolism. During intrauterine life, however, insulin is the most important hormone that regulates fetal growth. As insulin does not pass the placental barrier, the insulin found in fetal blood comes from the fetal pancreas. Fetal insulin is detected as early as weeks 8–9, although it remains relatively inactive until week 20, when an insulin response to glucose is evident[9]. An exogenous glucose response depends on fetal serum glucose levels, which regulate the sensitivity of pancreatic β cells[10]. Thus, chronic fetal hyperglycemia accelerates the development of mechanisms secreting insulin in such a way that newborns of diabetic mothers are predisposed to show a secretory insulin response similar to that of adults[11].

Insulin receptors in the fetal liver peak between weeks 19 and 25; however, the highest affinity to these receptors is reached at more advanced gestational ages[12].

Hyperinsulinemia promotes glucose storage in the form of glycogen, as well as lipolysis and uptake and use of amino acids. Experimental studies on the effect of insulin on fetal growth in rhesus monkeys have shown that insulin induces organomegaly, and an increase in fetal and placental weight as well as in crown–rump length[13]. The importance of insulin in fetal growth control is illustrated in clinical practice by the common finding of hyperinsulinemia in fetal macrosomia associated with maternal diabetes, Beckwith–Wiedemann syndrome or nesidioblastosis.

Insulin-like growth factors This group of peptides with structural similarities to the amino acid chain of proinsulin[14], and previously known as somatomedins, may act through endocrine, paracrine or autocrine mechanisms[15]. Insulin-like growth factors (IGF) promote fetal growth by the following mechanisms: glucose metabolism stimulation, DNA synthesis and cell proliferation. The two forms of circulating IGF, IGF factor-I (IGF-I) and IGF factor-II (IGF-II), are detectable at 13 weeks of gestation and do not pass the placental barrier. Fetal and maternal serum levels of IGF-I increase as pregnancy advances and correlate with fetal and placental weight[16], whereas a similar correlation has not been found for IGF-II and fetal weight. Amniotic fluid levels of IGF-II do not vary during pregnancy[17].

Two types of cellular receptors for IGF have been identified[18]. Type I receptors are similar to insulin receptors, whereas type II receptors are specific for IGF-II. In addition, two different binding proteins have also been recognized, although the exact mechanism of action of binding proteins is not well known.

Other hormones The effect of growth hormone on the normal fetus is minimal, with the liver being the only fetal tissue expressing growth hormone receptors. Similarly, the effect of other hormones on fetal growth is negligible.

Maternal and environmental factors

Some factors have empirically been associated with macrosomia, such as previous history of macrosomia, multiparity, maternal obesity, maternal age and maternal height, excessive weight gain during pregnancy, prolonged gestation and slow delivery[19–22].

A significant increase in the occurrence of macrosomia has been documented in women over the age of 35. Multiparous women – two or three previous pregnancies – have a significantly higher number of macrosomic infants. Maternal height has shown some influence when it is greater than 160 cm and especially when greater than 170 cm.

CLINICAL IMPLICATIONS

Excessive fetal weight is associated with a significant increase in perinatal morbidity and mortality. At delivery, the macrosomic fetus is more likely to suffer shoulder dystocia, traumatic injury and asphyxia (more common in pregnancies complicated by diabetes mellitus)[23,24]. In infants weighing more than 4000 g, shoulder dystocia occurs in 4.7–10% of cases. In the absence of maternal diabetes, the incidence of shoulder dystocia varies between 9.4% and 22.6% in infants weighing more than 4500 g[25,26].

Elective Cesarean section for the macrosomic fetus has been advocated by some authors in order to prevent complications, although others claim that macrosomic fetuses born by Cesarean section do not present a significantly different morbidity from those born by spontaneous delivery[27].

Macrosomia is observed in 50% of pregnancies complicated by insulin-dependent diabetes mellitus[23,24]. Macrosomia in infants from diabetic mothers is characterized by selective organomegaly, with increase in fat and muscle mass contributing to a disproportionately increased size of the trunk and shoulders. Brain size, however, remains unchanged and cephalic biomorphic data are within normal limits[28]. This condition has been named asymmetrical or partial macrosomia.

Although macrosomia has traditionally been related to maternal diabetes mellitus, only 2% of infants with macrosomia are born to diabetic mothers[29]. Other risk factors that probably account for the largest percentage of fetuses with macrosomia (called by some authors symmetrical or generalized macrosomia) include genetic factors, prolonged gestation, multiparity, maternal age (over 35 years) and excessive initial maternal weight[30].

Measurements of the subcutaneous fat and skin fold have demonstrated statistically significant increases in body fat in infants born to diabetic mothers as compared with newborns of non-diabetic mothers. Histopathological examination of fat tissue obtained by biopsy of the gluteal region has shown hypertrophy of adipocytes. Maternal serum glucose levels and fetal serum insulin levels have been correlated with hypertrophy of fat cells, which suggests that fetal subcutaneous fat accumulation may be an indicator of the quality of glycemic control during pregnancy[31–33].

References

1. McKeown T, Marshall T. Influences on fetal growth. *J Reprod Med* 1976;47:167
2. Kloosterman GJ. On intrauterine growth: the significance of prenatal care. *J Gynecol Obstet* 1970;8:895
3. Jones KL. Beckwith–Wiedemann syndrome. In *Smith's Recognizable Patterns of Human Malformation*, 4th edn. Philadelphia: Saunders, 1988
4. Beckwith JB. Macroglossia, omphalocele, adrenal cytomegaly, gigantism, and hyperplastic visceromegaly. *Birth Defects* 1969;5:188
5. Herzberg SA, Seyed S, Hill D. Possible etiologic mechanism for the overgrowth and hypo-glycemia in patients with Beckwith–Wiedemann syndrome. *Clin Res* 1979;27:812
6. Irving I. Exomphalos with macroglossia: a study of 11 cases. *J Pediatr Surg* 1967;2:499
7. Jones KL. Soto's syndrome. In *Smith's Recognizable Patterns of Human Malformation*, 4th edn. Philadelphia: Saunders, 1988
8. Weaver DD, Graham CB, Thomas IT, Smith DW. A new overgrowth syndrome with accelerated skeletal maturation, unusual facies and camptodactyly. *J Pediatr* 1974;84:547
9. Adam PAJ, Teramo K, Raiha N. Human fetal insulin metabolism early in gestation. Responses to acute elevation of the fetal glucose concentration and placental transfer of human insulin-I-131. *Diabetes* 1969;18:409
10. Fowden AL. Effects of arginine and glucose on the release of insulin in the sheep fetus. *J Endocrinol* 1980;87:113
11. Oakley NW, Beard RW, Turner RC. Effect of sustained maternal hyperglycemia on the fetus in normal and diabetic pregnancies. *Br Med J* 1972;8:466
12. Neufeld ND, Scott M, Kaplan SA. Ontogeny of the mammalian receptor. *Dev Biol* 1980;78:151
13. Susa JB, Schwartz R. Effects of hyperinsulinemia in the primate fetus. *Diabetes* 1985;34:36
14. Daughaday WH, Heath E. Physiological and possible clinical significance of epidermal and nerve growth factors. *J Clin Endocrinol Metab* 1984;13:207
15. D'Ercole AJ, Stiles AD, Underwood LE. Tissue concentrations of somatomedin C: further evidence of multiple sites of synthesis and paracrine/autocrine mechanisms of action. *Proc Natl Acad Sci USA* 1984;81:935
16. Gluckman PD, Barret-Johnson JJ, Butler JH. Studies of insulin like growth factor I and II by specific radioligand assays in umbilical cord blood. *Clin Endocrinol* 1983;19:405
17. Ashton IK, Zapf J, Einschenk J. Insulin-like growth factors (IGF) I and II in human fetal plasma and relationship to gestational age and fetal size during mid pregnancy. *Acta Endocrinol* 1985;10:558
18. Shigematsu K, Niwa M, Kurihara M. Receptor autoradiographic localization of insulin-like growth factor (IGF-I) binding sites in human fetal and adult adrenal glands. *Life Sci* 1985;46:383
19. Udall JN, Harrison GG, Vaucher Y. Interaction of maternal and neonatal obesity. *Pediatrics* 1978;62:17
20. Hansen JP. Older maternal age and pregnancy outcome: a review of the literature. *Obstet Gynecol Surv* 1986;41:726
21. Boyd ME, Usher RH, McLean FH, Kramer MS. Obstetric consequences of postmaturity. *Am J Obstet Gynecol* 1988;158:334
22. O'Leary JA. Preconceptual risk factors. In O'Leary JA, ed. *Shoulder Dystocia and Birth Injury*. New York: McGraw-Hill, 1992
23. Lavin JP, Lovelace DR, Miodovnik M, Knowles HC, Barden TP. Clinical experience with 107 diabetic pregnancies. *Am J Obstet Gynecol* 1983; 147:742–52
24. Sepe SJ, Connell FA, Geiss LS, Teutsch SM. Gestational diabetes: incidence, maternal characteristics, and perinatal outcome. *Diabetes* 1985;34(Suppl 2):13–16
25. Acker DB, Sachs BP, Friedman EA. Risk factors for shoulder dystocia. *Obstet Gynecol* 1985;66:762–8
26. Sandmire HF, O'Halloin TJ. Shoulder dystocia: its incidence and associated risk factors. *Int J Gynecol Obstet* 1988;26:65–73
27. Delpapa E, Mueller Heubach E. Pregnancy outcome following ultrasound diagnosis of macrosomia. *Obstet Gynecol* 1991;78:340–3
28. Mondanlou HD, Komatsu G, Dorchester W, Freeman RK, Bosu SK. Large-for-gestational age neonates: anthropometric reasons for shoulder dystocia. *Obstet Gynecol* 1982;60:417–23
29. Boyd ME, Usher RH, McLean FH. Fetal macrosomia: prediction, risks, proposed management. *Obstet Gynecol* 1983;61:715–22
30. Spellacy WN, Miller S, Winegar A, Peterson PQ. Macrosomia: maternal characteristics and infant complications. *Obstet Gynecol* 1985;66:158–61
31. Brans YW, Shannon DL, Hunter MA. Maternal diabetes and neonatal macrosomia. II. Neonatal anthropometric measurements. *Early Hum Dev* 1983;8:297–305
32. Enzi G, Inelmen EM, Caretta F, Villani F, Zanardo U, Debiasi F. Development of adipose tissue in newborns of gestational diabetic and insulin-dependent mothers. *Diabetes* 1980;29:100–4
33. Whitelaw A. Subcutaneous fat in newborn infants of diabetic mothers. *Lancet* 1977;1:15–18

Diagnosis of fetal macrosomia　8

J. M. Carrera, M. Torrents and A. Muñoz

INTRODUCTION

Although fetal macrosomia can be suspected by ultrasound examination relatively early during pregnancy, it is usually detected at the beginning of the third trimester. Sonographic prediction of fetal weight based on weight estimation equations is associated with a 3–4% overestimation. The reliability of these methods has been questioned by some authors[1–4]. Probably the most frequent cause of fetal weight overestimation lies in the fact that equations are designed for fetuses with normal body composition; macrosomic fetuses and more often, fetuses in diabetic pregnancies, have a high percentage of fat tissue, which has a lower density than that of muscle tissue[5]. For this reason, fetal weight estimation during the second trimester of pregnancy is considered to be more sensitive than weight estimation in the third trimester.

CEPHALIC BIOMETRIC MEASUREMENTS FOR THE ESTIMATION OF FETAL WEIGHT

When the measurement of the biparietal diameter is above 2 SD, fetal macrosomia can be predicted in 7–96% of cases[6–11]. Most authors, however, have indicated that the prediction of fetal weight by measuring biparietal diameter has a low sensitivity, which is even lower in fetuses from diabetic mothers in whom the growth pattern of biparietal diameter is usually within the normal range[12].

ABDOMINAL BIOMETRIC MEASUREMENTS FOR THE ESTIMATION OF FETAL WEIGHT

Abdominal biometric studies seem to be the most efficient parameter for predicting

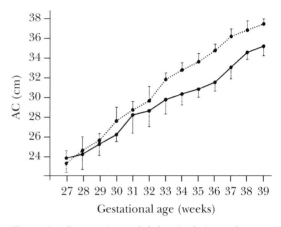

Figure 1 Comparison of abdominal circumference (AC) growth curves in large-for-gestational-age (dotted line) fetuses from diabetic mothers and appropriate-for-dates (unbroken line) fetuses. The acceleration in the growth rate of the abdominal circumference clearly begins from 32 weeks in the large-for-gestational-age fetuses. From reference 11

macrosomia. More than 50% of fetuses from women with gestational diabetes show abdominal diameters above the 95th centile. Landon and colleagues[11] showed that fetuses from diabetic mothers clearly departed from appropriate-for-dates fetuses at week 32 – the time at which marked acceleration in the growth rate of the abdominal circumference begins (Figure 1). In fact, measurement of the abdominal circumference alone during the third trimester of pregnancy is a useful parameter to make the diagnosis of fetal macrosomia. Tamura and co-workers[9] diagnosed 78% of large-for-dates fetuses when the abdominal circumference was above the 90th centile in the 2 weeks before labor. Bochner and associates[13] identified 87% of macrosomic fetuses in diabetic pregnancies when the abdominal circumference was above

Table 1 Sensitivity, specificity and predictive value of the femur length/abdominal circumference index for the diagnosis of macrosomia in fetuses from diabetic mothers. From reference 16

Point of intersection	Sensitivity	Specificity	PPV	NPV
20.0	0.64	0.60	0.36	0.83
19.8	0.58	0.65	0.37	0.81
19.6	0.53	0.69	0.38	0.81
19.4	0.48	0.74	0.42	0.80
19.2	0.42	0.77	0.39	0.79

PPV, positive predicitve value; NPV, negative predictive value

the 90th centile at 30–33 weeks of gestation, although false-positive results occurred in up to 14% of cases. On the other hand, the negative predictive value of a normal abdominal circumference (below the 90th centile) is 96.4%.

BIOMETRIC INDICES

It is well known that head/abdominal circumference or area ratio varies during pregnancy, i.e. > 1 up to 35 weeks' gestation, equal to 1 at 35–36 weeks and < 1 from week 36 until delivery. Although this parameter is generally used to diagnose asymmetrical intrauterine growth restriction in fetuses with asymmetric macrosomia, this ratio decreases due to an exaggerated growth of the abdomen[14]. In a study carried out by our group, it was found that in macrosomic fetuses this ratio was already equal to 1 at 30 weeks' gestation.

Murata and Martin[8] and Wladimiroff and Bloemsma[6] found that the ratio between biparietal and thoracic diameters was below the 5th centile in 53% of fetuses with accelerated growth as opposed to only 2% in normally developed fetuses. Elliot and colleagues[15] diagnosed 87% of fetuses weighing more than 4000 g when there was a difference of ≥ 1.4 cm between thoracic and biparietal diameters.

Indices based on two fetal biometrical parameters, independently of gestational age, are used by some authors for the diagnosis of macrosomia. These methods are similar to the neonatal weight index used by pediatricians. Hadlock and co-workers[14] used a weight index (femur length/abdominal circumference × 100) that in normal fetuses was 22 ± 2 but in macrosomic fetuses decreased to 20.5 ± 2, with a sensitivity of 63% and a specificity of 86%. However, Benson and associates[16] demonstrated that the sensitivity of this parameter for the diagnosis of macrosomia in fetuses from diabetic mothers was low (Table 1). In the study of Bracero and colleagues[17], when the mean abdominal diameter/femur length ratio was greater than 1.385 macrosomic fetuses from diabetic mothers were detected with a diagnostic sensitivity of 79% and a specificity of 80%.

Statistically significant results in the comparison of some parameters between appropriate-for-dates and macrosomic fetuses as well as macrosomic fetuses and normally developed fetuses from diabetic mothers are shown in Tables 2 and 3.

SERIAL ULTRASONOGRAPHIC CONTROL OF FETAL GROWTH

It seems evident that a serial ultrasonographic assessment of fetal growth is more useful for predicting anomalies of fetal growth than a single echographic study, even if such a study is performed immediately before childbirth.

Abdominal fetal growth of ≥ 1.2 cm per week or an accelerated increase of this parameter at 32 weeks' gestation suggests fetal macrosomia, with a sensitivity of 84% and a specificity of 85%[11]. In a serial echographic

Table 2 Comparison of fetal parameters between large-for-gestational-age (LGA)fetuses and appropriate-for-dates (AGD) fetuses. From reference 14

Parameter	AGD group (mean ± SD)	LGA group (mean ± SD)	p Value
BPD (cm)	9.2 ± 0.4	9.6 ± 0.4	< 0.0001
CC (cm)	33.7 ± 1.1	35.2 ± 1.3	< 0.0001
AC (cm)	33.6 ± 1.6	37.4 ± 1.3	< 0.0001
FL (cm)	7.4 ± 0.4	7.6 ± 0.3	< 0.0001
CC/AC ratio	1.0 ± 0.05	0.94 ± 0.04	< 0.0001
FL/AC*	22.0 ± 1.0	20.5 ± 1.0	< 0.0001

BPD, biparietal diameter; CC, cephalic circumference; AC, abdominal circumference; FL, femur length; *expressed as FL/AC × 100

Table 3 Comparison of selected biometrical fetal parameters in macrosomic fetuses from diabetic and non-diabetic mothers. From reference 14

Parameter	LGA fetuses from non-diabetic mothers (n = 9) (mean ± SD)	AGD fetuses diabetic mothers (n = 9) (mean ± SD)	p Value
BPD (cm)	9.65 ± 0.4	9.54 ± 0.4	> 0.05
CC (cm)	35.22 ± 1.3	34.96 ± 1.4	> 0.05
AC (cm)	37.30 ± 1.4	37.78 ± 0.5	> 0.05
FL (cm)	7.68 ± 0.3	7.40 ± 0.5	> 0.05
CC/AC ratio	0.95 ± 0.04	0.93 ± 0.03	> 0.05
FL/AC†	22.7 ± 1.1	19.6 ± 1.2	< 0.05*
Weight at birth (g)	4307 ± 271	4237 ± 228	> 0.05

LGA, large-for-gestational-age; AGD, appropriate-for-dates; BPD, biparietal diameter; CC, cephalic circumference; AC, abdominal circumference; FL, femur length; *statistically significant; †expressed as FL/AC × 100

study of 23 children from diabetic mothers, Ogata and colleagues[12] found that in ten of them the abdominal circumference at 28 and 32 weeks' gestation was higher than the expected value, with increased subcutaneous tissue thickness and increased insulin levels in the amniotic fluid.

ULTRASONOGRAPHIC MEASUREMENT OF SUBCUTANEOUS TISSUE THICKNESS

Neonatal studies have shown a good correlation between skinfold thickness and birth weight, although with quite a large error range[18]. According to this finding, some authors have suggested the use of subcutaneous tissue thickness for the detection of accelerated fetal growth.

During the first 6 months of pregnancy, deposition of fat in the subcutaneous tissue is scarce, but from 28 to 40 weeks' gestation the percentage of fat of the total fetal weight increased from 4 to 14%[19]. Vaucher and colleagues[18] showed that, between 24 and 41 weeks' gestation, the subcutaneous tissue thickness in the mid-biceps, triceps and abdomen (at 2 cm from the umbilical cord insertion) was 1–3.4 mm. According to Hill and associates[20] subcutaneous tissue thickness in the mid-calf, thigh and abdomen increased from 1 mm at week 15 of gestation to 5.5 mm in the fetus at term. At the end of pregnancy, approximately 75% of body fat was found in the subcutaneous tissue[21].

Some authors have shown that, in cases of intrauterine growth restriction, there is a decrease in the subcutaneous tissue thickness as a result of a reduction of body fat[19,22,23]. However, the relative dispersion of normal values both in fetal and in neonatal studies indicates that the measurement of this parameter has a low sensitivity for the detection of intrauterine growth restriction[23]. The study of Hill and co-workers[20] also confirms the low sensitivity of this parameter for the differentiation of large- from appropriate-for-gestational-age fetuses.

Subcutaneous fat and muscular tissues are indirect indicators of caloric and protein stores of the fetus. Neonates with large muscular stores and limited fat reservoirs have a higher weight than neonates with much fat and a poor muscular mass[24], because of the low density of the fat tissue as compared with the muscles. This occurs, for example, in infants born from heavy smokers in whom a decreased birth weight is related to reduction of muscular mass, the fat tissue remaining unaffected. For this reason, the assessment of subcutaneous tissue thickness alone does not seem useful for detecting fetal growth anomalies.

MEASUREMENT OF THE AMNIOTIC FLUID VOLUME

A relationship between fetal weight and amniotic fluid volume has been suggested[25,26]. The incidence of polyhydramnios is higher in pregnancies with large-for-gestational-age fetuses from non-diabetic women (17%) than in pregnancies with normal fetuses (8%); in contrast, oligohydramnios is less frequent in large-for-gestational-age fetuses (3%) than in fetuses of normal weight (9%)[27].

In the study of Benson and associates[27], a macrosomic fetus is excluded in the presence of oligohydramnios and an estimated fetal weight below the 90th centile, whereas the evidence of polyhydramnios together with an estimated fetal weight above the 90th centile increases the possibility of fetal macrosomia.

PREDICTION OF FETAL WEIGHT BY OTHER TECHNIQUES

Fetal weight has been assessed by means of computed tomography (CT) and magnetic resonance imaging (MRI) in diabetic pregnancies. CT is used for measuring the width of fetal shoulders 48 h before childbirth. When this parameter is ≥ 14 cm a fetal weight greater than 4200 g is predicted with a sensitivity of 100% and a specificity of 87%[28].

With the use of MRI it is possible to determine the amount of subcutaneous tissue, which appears as a white linear image surrounding the whole fetal body.

References

1. Miller JM, Korndorfer FA III, Gabert HA. Fetal weight estimates in late pregnancy with emphasis on macrosomia. *J Clin Ultrasound* 1986;14:437–42
2. Benson CB, Doubilet PM, Satzman DH. Sonographic determination of fetal weight in diabetic pregnancy. *Am J Obstet Gynecol* 1987;156:441–4
3. Sabbagha RE, Minogue J, Tamura RK, Hungerford SA. Estimation of birth weight by use of ultrasonographic formulas targeted to large-, appropiate-, and small-for-gestational-age fetuses. *Am J Obstet Gynecol* 1989;160:854–60, discussion 860–2
4. Hirata GI, Medearis AL, Horenstein J, Bear MB, Flatt LD. Ultrasonographic estimation of fetal weight in the clinically macrosomic fetus. *Am J Obstet Gynecol* 1990;162:238–42

5. Bernstein JM, Catalano PM. Influence of fetal fat on the ultrasound estimation of fetal weight in diabetic mothers. *Obstet Gynecol* 1992;79:561–3

6. Wladimiroff J, Bloemsma FM. Ultrasonic diagnosis of the large-for-dates infant. *Obstet Gynecol* 1978;52:285–8

7. Crane JP, Kopta MM, Welt SI, Sauvage JP. Abnormal fetal growth patterns: ultrasonic diagnosis and management. *Obstet Gynecol* 1977;50:205–11

8. Murata Y, Martin CB Jr. Growth of the biparietal diameter of the fetal head in diabetic pregnancy. *Am J Obstet Gynecol* 1973;115:252–6

9. Tamura RK, Sabbagha RE, Depp R, Dooley SL, Socor Ml. Diabetic macrosomia: accuracy of third trimester ultrasound. *Obstet Gynecol* 1986;67:828–32

10. Naeye RL. The newborn infant of the diabetic mother. *Pa Med* 1968;75:69–72

11. Landon MB, Mintz M, Gabbe SG. Sonographic evaluation of fetal abdominal growth: predictor of the LGA infant in pregnancies complicated by diabetes mellitus. *Am J Obstet Gynecol* 1989;160:115–21

12. Ogata ES, Sabbagha R, Metzger BE, Pheps RL, Deep R, Freinkel N. Serial ultrasonography to asses evolving macrosomia: studies in 23 diabetic women. *J Am Med Assoc* 1980;243:2405–8

13. Bochner C, Meadanis AL, William J, Castro L, Hobel CJ, Wade ME. Early third trimester ultrasound screening in gestational diabetes to determine the risk of macrosomia and labor dystocia at term. *Am J Obstet Gynecol* 1987;157:703–8

14. Hadlock FP, Harrist RB, Fearneyhough R, Deter RL, Bark SK, Rossavik IK. Use of femur length/abdominal circumference ratio in detecting the macrosomic fetus. *Radiology* 1985;154:503–5

15. Elliot JP, Garite TJ, Freeman RK, McQuonn DS, Patel OM. Ultrasonic prediction of fetal macrosomia in diabetic patients. *Obstet Gynecol* 1982;60:159–62

16. Benson CB, Doubilet PM, Saltzman DH, Greene MF, Jones TB. Femur length/abdominal circumference ratio: poor predictor of macrosomic fetuses in diabetic mothers. *J Ultrasound Med* 1986;5:141

17. Bracero LA, Baxi Lu, Rey HR, Yeh MN. Use of ultrasound in antenatal diagnosis of large-for-gestational age infants in diabetic gravid patients. *Am J Obstet Gynecol* 1985;152:43–7

18. Vaucher YE, Harrison GG, Udall JN, Morrow G. Skinfold thickness in North American infants 24–41 weeks' gestation. *Hum Biol* 1984;56:713–31

19. Widdowson EM. Body composition of the fetus and infant. In Vesser HKA, ed. *Nutrition and Metabolism of the Fetus and Infant.* The Hague: Martinus Nijhoff Publishers, 1979:169–77

20. Hill LM, Guzick D, Boyles D, Merorino C, Ballone A, Gmiter P. Subcutaneous tissue thickness cannot be used to distinguish abnormalities of fetal growth. *Obstet Gynecol* 1992;80:268–71

21. Dauncey MJ, Gandy G, Gairdner D. Assessment of total body fat in infancy from skinfold thickness measurements. *Arch Dis Child* 1977;52:223–7

22. McLean F, Usher R. Measurements of liveborn fetal malnutrition infants compared with similar gestation and with similar birth-weight normal controls. *Biol Neonate* 1970;16:215–21

23. Brans YW, Sumners JE, Dweck HS, Cassady G. A noninvasive approach to body composition in the neonate: dynamic skinfold measurements. *Pediatr Res* 1974;8:215–22

24. Frisancho AR, Klayman JE, Matts J. Newborn body composition and its relationship to linear growth. *Am J Clin Nutr* 1977;30:704–74

25. Chamberlain PF, Manning PA, Morrison I, Harman CR, Lange IR. Ultrasound evaluation of amniotic fluid volume. *Am J Obstet Gynecol* 1984;150:250–4

26. Varma TR, Bateman S, Patel RH, Chamberlain GV, Pillai U. The relationship of increased amniotic fluid volume to perinatal outcome. *Int J Gynecol Obstet* 1988;27:327–33

27. Benson CB, Coughlin BF, Doubilet PM. Amniotic fluid volume in large-for-gestational-age fetuses of nondiabetic mothers. *J Ultrasound Med* 1991;10:149–51

28. Kitzmiller JL, Mall JC, Gin GD, Hendricks SK, Newman RB, Scheerer L. Measurement of fetal shoulder width with computed tomography in diabetic women. *Obstet Gynecol* 1987;70:941–5

Index